MW01068216

ESSENTIAL
FASTING

DI Books by Jordan Rubin and Josh Axe

The Beginner's Guide to Essential Oils

Essential Oils

DI Books by Jordan Rubin

Patient Heal Thyself

Planet Heal Thyself

Maker's Diet Meals

The Maker's Diet

The Joseph Blessing

Re-size America

The Maker's Diet Revolution

JORDAN RUBIN
AND DR. JOSH AXE

ESSENTIAL
FASTING

12 BENEFITS OF INTERMITTENT FASTING
& OTHER FASTING PLANS FOR ACCELERATING WEIGHT LOSS, CRUSHING CRAVINGS, AND REVERSING AGING

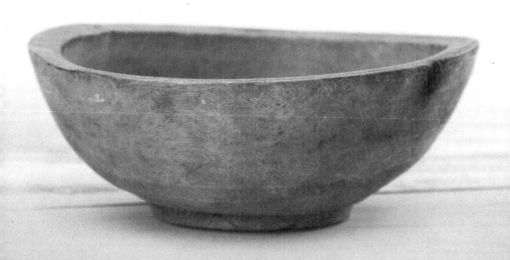

DESTINY IMAGE® PUBLISHERS, INC.
P.O. Box 310, Shippensburg, PA 17257-0310
"Promoting Inspired Lives."

This book and all other Destiny Image and Destiny Image Fiction books are available at Christian bookstores and distributors worldwide.

Cover design by Eileen Rockwell.

For more information on foreign distributors, call 717-532-3040.

Reach us on the Internet: www.destinyimage.com.

ISBN 13 TP: 978-0-7684-5475-8

ISBN 13 eBook: 978-0-7684-5473-4

ISBN 13 HC: 978-0-7684-5472-7

ISBN 13 LP: 978-0-7684-5474-1

For Worldwide Distribution, Printed in the U.S.A.

1 2 3 4 5 6 7 8 / 24 23 22 21 20

Contents

Part 3:

THE WHY BEHIND FASTING

Part 4:

HOW AND WHEN TO FAST

Part 5:

Part 6:
SMART FASTING TOOLS

PART 1

FASTING IS NOT A FAD

The History and Significance of Fasting

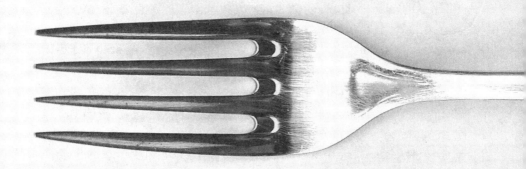

When Did Food Become the Enemy?

Modern life revolves around eating.

From family gatherings and date nights to holidays and religious celebrations, eating is always involved—and in most cases, food is the centerpiece of the event.

July 4th wouldn't be Independence Day without burgers and brats and hot dogs and chips and watermelon and ice cream and more. Thanksgiving is as much about what goes into our mouths as it is about family and thankfulness.

When we gather, we expect someone to be serving up something tasty.

Food is also a source of comfort. It can provide solace when stressed and a satisfying way to pass the time when bored. People eat when they are thirsty and when they are tired. People eat out of habit. People eat because of social pressure.

While none of this is technically wrong or anything to be ashamed of, it *is* indicative of modern society. Once upon a time, not that long ago in the context of life on earth, humanity ate only when necessary. There were no snacks in between lunch and dinner or late-night fourth meals. Dessert wasn't a given after every single meal.

It wasn't even until the turn of the twentieth century—thanks to the advent of grocery stores—that Americans gained 24/7 access to every kind of food imaginable at any time they desire, day or night.

In biblical times, and according to Exodus 16:12, there were two meals: one in the morning and one in the evening. Breakfast consisted of light fare in the early morning hours that included bread, fruits, and cheese. This meal was intended as fuel for hours of backbreaking toil and labor (or forty years of wandering in the desert). Dinner was the more substantial spread of the two that likely contained a protein source such as meat.

It is also interesting to note that the Bible is not short on references to food. From Genesis to Revelation, God continually reveals the importance of food. In fact, in the gospels alone, food is mentioned at least ninety times, and eating is mentioned over 100 times.

God designed us to eat!

What He did *not* design us for was to eat *past* the feeling of satiety. He did not create us to eat when we are not hungry or eat because we are bored or stressed. He did not design us to fill up on nutritionally empty foods and sugary drinks that cause dysfunction in the body. God also did not plan for us to eat around the clock.

God designed us to eat!

As much as we were designed to eat, we were *also designed* to fast.

Your body already does it every single night. That's why breakfast is made of the words *break* and *fast*, because that is what eating after a period of no food does. It breaks a period of fasting. What we've gotten wrong is how *long* to abstain from food each day.

Because of modern eating habits, America now faces significant problems. The obesity epidemic alone is linked to almost every major lifestyle disease and leading mortality causes in our country.

Prolonged overconsumption of food (particularly processed food) is linked to weight gain, acne, shortness of breath, headaches, depression, significantly increased risk of heart attack and stroke, high cholesterol, bloating and puffiness, mental fogginess, high blood pressure, insulin resistance leading to type 2 diabetes, and dental distress.

In other words, too much food is killing us.

It wasn't supposed to be like this. The human body is a remarkable machine designed to turn food into fuel that powers our brains, our hearts, our movements, and every single other function—from giving us the energy to run a marathon to healing the body at the cellular level.

It's easy to see why our ancestors believed that the gods controlled their health. Without microscopes and the intricate knowledge of science and nutrition that we have today, how would we imagine our bodies can breathe, function, and heal? To the people of antiquity, it must have indeed seemed supernatural.

Thanks to the wealth of scientific discovery, we now know precisely how the human body functions. We can follow a morsel of food from the time it enters our mouth, and we understand the path it takes, how it breaks down, what it contains, and how its contents affect every cell in our bodies. That is precisely why food is so important. It shapes life itself.

Unfortunately, that power works both ways.

The wrong food and too much of it can also destroy our bodies. Nothing more clearly explains why our health is in the severe jeopardy it is in today.

Food serves as far more than just the means to keep us alive and provide us with nutrients—and it is that very fact that makes this topic so complex. If humans merely consumed food according to the "eat to live" philosophy, we'd all be laser-focused solely on taking in foods that bring health and vitality to our bodies.

The problem is most people "live to eat." We are also in a big hurry all the time. Fast-food signs serve as beacons of relief on the way home from the office after a long day, offering an instant family dinner for under twenty dollars. We've become wired to equate food with fun, family, friendship, and familiarity. We've also come to expect meals to be overly salty, fatty, sweet, and convenient.

On the other hand, society tells us that being obese, overweight, or even just a "normal" size is unattractive. We are fat-shamed by images on the screen, in advertisements, and on social media of paper-thin women and men with chiseled physiques.

These conflicting messages have left us with unsatisfying solutions for balancing when and what to eat with our hectic lives. To many, the word *diet* itself represents taking away the joy of eating. Others end up in a never-ending cycle of yo-yo dieting, jumping from one fad crash diet to the next.

Add the word *fasting* into the mix, and you'll send plenty of people running as quickly as they can in the other direction as words such as *starving*, *hungry*, and *dangerous* often come to mind.

It's a mess. If we want to fix it, we must strip away our preconceived notions of what food represents and what fasting is and is not, and then arm ourselves with strategies that produce results based on specific goals.

And believe us when we say that fasting is one of the *best* ways to achieve almost any health goal. If you want to lose weight, burn fat, cleanse and detox your body, boost your energy, lift brain fog, and reverse disease, you need to be fasting.

Fasting has also been clinically studied and shown to relieve arthritis, reduce skin problems, shrink tumors, and help with addictions to food.[1] Yes, bondage can be broken from food addictions that have limited your life for far too long.

If you're thinking, "I can't fast because I don't want to give up food" or "I can't fast because of my condition," then take heart. We promise there is a fast discussed in this book that is right for you.

We are not going to tell you that the only fasting option is to go without food and to drink only water. Although that is one type of fast, there are many different varieties—some are more challenging, and some are surprisingly easy to implement.

Fasting could very well create the breakthrough you've been searching for.

Just be prepared because this could very well create the breakthrough you've been searching for.

If you struggle with digestive issues, you will be amazed at how much better your gut functions when you implement fasting.

If you are battling a disease such as cancer or an autoimmune disease, fasting can dramatically change the direction of your life.

If you've tried different diets and supplements but have simply not experienced the weight loss or energy increase you desired, fasting could very well be the key to breakthrough.

The best part about this powerful health tool is that unlike expensive diet plans and programs, fasting is free!

And who doesn't want to be healed at no cost?

We can't wait to help guide you on this journey. So let's start by discussing the history of fasting to understand how long fasting has been a part of the human experience.

The Ancient Origins of Fasting

There are thousands of resources, books, and programs available on fasting today. It seems to be the newest and hottest trend in health and fitness.

As the saying goes, "There is nothing new, except what has been forgotten." Fasting is no new trend. It's been hiding in plain sight all along.

Not anymore!

Fasting has always brought strength and power, but the reason more people don't utilize it even today might be because fasting is intimidating. It can also be incredibly challenging to abstain from food for longer than you usually would. Practicing self-control and resisting the urge to eat when it's been a few hours since your last meal is not the norm in our society. Today's culture is all about instant gratification. Fasting represents a denial of fleshly cravings, and that's a tough concept to sell in America.

So perhaps if more people understood just how long fasting has been in use and why, it would help them make the conscious decision to try this time-tested ancient tradition.

At this point in your health journey, you have probably figured out that there are no quick fixes. There are no magic pills. There is no such thing as a diet or workout program that allows you to eat whatever you want whenever you want and still lose weight and feel better.

The silver bullet for health and weight loss? It just doesn't exist.

The sooner we collectively come to terms with that, the sooner we can start finding real and proven ways to feel and look better.

Instead of searching for that silver bullet, more people now realize that the ancient healing traditions of the past hold the answers we need.

Hippocrates (460–370 BC) is often called the father of modern medicine. It is interesting to note that among the treatments he prescribed was fasting. Hippocrates wrote, "To eat when you are sick is to feed your illness."[2] It feels strange that we refer to Hippocrates as the father of modern medicine when you consider the fact that what he practiced didn't look anything like Western medicine practiced today. Two of his most significant prescriptions for health were fasting and sunbathing.

Greek historian and writer Plutarch also echoed these sentiments when he wrote, "Instead of using medicine, better fast today."[3] Two other Ancient Greek thinkers, Plato and Aristotle, were also staunch supporters of fasting.

The ancient Greeks believed that the best medical treatment could be found through nature—both *in* it and by *observing* it. If you have ever watched a sick animal, you may have noticed that it does not eat when it becomes critically ill. Humans have a similar response, which is why so many illnesses are accompanied by loss of appetite as one of the most common symptoms.

For this reason, fasting has long been known as evoking the "physician within."

> Fasting has long been known as evoking the "physician within."

This instinct to fast is undoubtedly familiar to anyone who has ever had the flu. Remember the last time you were sick with a severe viral infection? If you are like most people, you had no desire to eat.

You've probably heard the phrase, "Starve a fever." This is because when your body is fighting an illness, the last thing it wants to do is have to deal with digesting a hamburger or doughnuts as well.

The ancient Greeks also believed that fasting improves cognitive abilities. Think about last year's big Thanksgiving meal. When you gorge on turkey, stuffing, sweet potatoes, and pumpkin pie, do you feel more energetic and mentally alert afterward? Of course not.

A nap is usually what immediately follows such a large meal. One of the reasons why is because your body sends more blood to your digestive system to cope with the massive influx of food, leaving less blood going to the brain.

The Greeks were not the only ones who recognized the tremendous benefits of fasting. The founder of toxicology and another major influencer of modern Western medicine, Paracelsus, wrote, "Fasting is the greatest remedy, the physician within."[4]

Additionally, practitioners of ancient healing systems such as Ayurveda and Chinese medicine discovered that planning regular fasts could impact mental clarity, emotional stability, and overall wellness.

One of America's founding fathers Benjamin Franklin (1706–1790) once wrote, "The best of all medicines is resting and fasting."[5]

Fasting for spiritual purposes has been a longtime mainstay in virtually every major religion in the world. In a religious context, fasting is often called *cleansing* or *purification*, but it essentially amounts to the same thing. Three founders of the world's major religions (Jesus, Buddha, and Muhammad) all agreed that fasting is beneficial.

Fasting developed from the earliest recorded times as something that was intrinsically beneficial to not only the spirit but also to the body.

Fasting is a tradition that has weathered the test of time. If this were a harmful practice, it would not have been utilized and promoted by some of the most prominent figures in history and medicine.

Fasting in the Bible

We believe that more than anything else, fasting is about unlocking the healer within in order for you to experience a genuine breakthrough.

When we say *breakthrough*, we are talking about catapulting your life to an entirely new level—not a tiptoe, not even a walk to the next line, but a genuine transformation where strongholds are removed, and you can finally get your health where it needs to be.

You can accomplish all of this through fasting—the not-so-hidden secret from the Bible that has been largely forgotten in modern times until recently.

The early church fathers, Luther, Calvin, and Wesley all practiced this health "secret." It was one practiced by the great men and women of God, from Moses, David, and Solomon to Daniel, Esther, and Jesus Himself.

According to the prehistoric Germanic etymology of the word we know today as *fasting*, the original meaning was "to hold firmly" and evolved into the idea of "having firm control of oneself."

To us, that is incredibly accurate, because when you fast, you take control—control over your own body and over food addictions and habits that may have led you down the path to dysfunction and disease.

In writing this book, it dawned on us that sin came into this world through our appetite. In other words, it originated in the lust of food. Eve saw the fruit of the tree of the knowledge of good and evil and wanted a taste. She and Adam had access to the purest, most amazing food on Earth, but all she wanted was the one thing she couldn't have. The forbidden fruit appealed to Eve's eye, and

When you fast, you take control over your own body and over food addictions and habits that may have led you down the path to dysfunction and disease.

she and Adam ate—and sin entered the world due to giving in to those appetites.

It was the only thing in their perfect utopia she could not consume, but she just couldn't resist.

Remember Esau? He was willing to give away his birthright for a meal. Food is just that powerful. Esau was simply giving in to the primal desire we all feel to satisfy hunger and therefore stay alive.

Thankfully, thousands of years later, Jesus showed us that man could resist the desires of the physical body in order to achieve great things. He started His ministry after forty days without consuming any food.

Jesus was all man and all God, but in this case, there is no reason to believe this was a supernatural fast. Biblical scholars believe that Jesus didn't eat, but He drank water during that time. Why? Because you can go without food for months and survive. However, you can go without water for only three to four days. At the end of those forty days, the Word says that "Jesus was hungry," but it didn't say He was thirsty.

During His fast, satan came to Him and said, *"If You are the Son of God, command that these stones become bread"* (Matt. 4:3) Jesus was weak. Jesus was hungry. But He said, *"Man shall not live by bread alone, but by every word that proceeds from the mouth of God"* (v. 4).

Jesus didn't consume food, but He still "ate." He *feasted* on the Word of God, and that sustained Him during those forty days. Jesus prepared for the ministry of salvation, the ministry of reconciliation by abasing and emptying Himself and going without solid food.

Fasting can do things in your life that no other health practice can. That's why for thousands of years great men and women of God have fasted, and that's also why your breakthrough is only a fast away.

Fasting can do things in
your life that no other
health practice can.

THREE BIBLICAL FASTS

There are three types of fast mentioned in the Bible. The first is a *standard* or *normal fast*. This fast would be defined as consuming no food but drinking water. When we look throughout Scripture, we conclude that a "normal fast" would have been a water-only fast. This is the fast that Jesus likely undertook for forty days.

A standard or normal fast is simple, yet also incredibly difficult. That is also why it produces impressive results that we'll talk about later.

The second type of fasts in the Bible is an *absolute fast*, which means consuming no food or water. Every year, the people of Israel are commanded to fast on one day called Yom Kippur, also known as the Day of Atonement. They neither eat nor drink. Esther declared an absolute fast when Haman, the enemy of the Jews, was about to destroy her entire people, and Moses completed a forty-day absolute fast.

Never in Scripture was an absolute fast done for more than three days except by Moses. Scholars believe this means that when Moses was in the presence of God, he was supernaturally able to consume no water or food because humans can't survive more than a few days without water.

We don't *ever* recommend absolute fasting (also called dry fasting) to anyone. We will not be discussing it in this book because it's simply not a good idea for most people, but it is worth noting that it was a form of fasting mentioned in the Bible and in some parts of the world is still practiced today for religious reasons.

Finally, there's the *partial fast*. The partial fast is typified by a cleanse or fast popularly known as the *Daniel fast*. Daniel went on two fasts—one that was ten days and one that was twenty-one days. During both, he avoided certain things and ate others.

If you've never heard of the Daniel fast, rest assured we will discuss it in greater detail later in the book and explain how to do the Daniel fast yourself safely. In addition to the Daniel fast, we will cover numerous other types of fasts and cleanses designed to bring healing into your life and help you regain control of your mind, your body, and your decisions.

Get Ready for Breakthrough

Whether you are a fasting novice and nervous about how your body will react or you have been fasting for years, there is a fasting type that works for everyone. Get ready to learn more about each type as we explore the many benefits of fasting, the pitfalls, and the best practices, as well as supplements and other tips that can turn fasting from an intimidating mystery into a routine and powerful practice in your life.

As much as we'll talk about fasting in this book, it's important to note that the Bible also recognizes eating and its tremendous importance. Food is and will always be a central part of our lives.

As we discussed at the start of this book, food signifies celebration. It provides an opportunity to share not only food but also conversation. We fellowship and grow closer to others over a meal. Eating is a sign of contentment and provides a satisfying way to relax.

It's crucial that you understand how much we love food too! Finding delicious new recipes and breaking bread with our families is one of the great highlights of every day for us. That is why we also provide our recommendations for the best and most delicious foods to consume when you are *not* fasting.

In life, there's always a balance.

We're not expecting you to give up Thanksgiving or stop eating all the foods you love. What we are saying is that fasting will open doors for you that have remained closed for far too long. Fasting will show you just how strong you are and just how much control you have over your health. Fasting will help you appreciate food in new and exciting ways!

No man knows the day or hour he will pass from this earth. That is not in our control. What is in our control is how well we live out the days we are given. Use fasting as a tool to get the most out of every day you have.

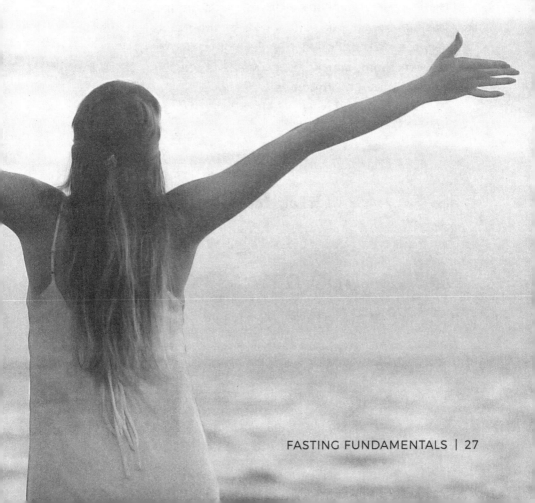

PART 2

FASTING FUNDAMENTALS

Basics, Definitions, and Types of Fasting

Not **What** but **When** to Eat

Fasting is a *natural* discipline that brings about a *supernatural* breakthrough. We wholeheartedly believe that by making fasting a part of your eating philosophy, you will experience a breakthrough in your life and your health.

Think about it—without even knowing about the scientifically proven health benefits that we will discuss in greater detail a little later in the book, nearly every religious group throughout history has practiced some variation of fasting rituals. Yet, whenever you hear fasting mentioned, there is a great deal of hesitation and doubt, even today, as the fasting craze is sweeping through the health and fitness communities.

Fasting is a *natural* discipline that brings about a *supernatural* breakthrough.

The issue could very well be that when people think of the word *fasting*, the term *starving* also comes to mind.

It's essential to set the record straight before we go any further. Fasting and starving are two different things. Starving is the *involuntary* absence of food. In the traditional sense of the word, starving is not something deliberate or within a person's control to stop. On the other hand, fasting is the *voluntary* withholding of food for spiritual, health, or other reasons.

Another key difference is that starving is usually prolonged and takes place after an extended period of consistently (but not purposefully) not getting enough food. Fasting is something you decide to do for some time, from a few hours to months. And in many cases, fasting does not involve going for more than a day without consuming food.

We like to think of fasting as a way of life, not a fad, a trend, or a "thing" that you do once and then stop. When you adjust your mindset and accept that fasting is already a part of your life, whether you realize it or not (you fast every time you go to sleep at night), it makes the subject much more approachable. It also makes integrating it into your routine far more feasible.

So the pertinent issue now becomes, "*When* exactly should I be eating each day?"

Until recently no one questioned the ingrained idea that breakfast is the most important meal. The issue with that idea, however, comes down to biology and is not as simple to defend as breakfast proponents wish.

While it is true that some foods are better than others, all foods promote an insulin response. This fact is especially important to understand in the age of insulin resistance and type 2 diabetes in which we live. When it comes to the worst offenders, starchy carbohydrates (bread, chips, processed food, french fries, etc.) and sugary foods such as cookies and pastries rank at the top. Even protein in the form of organic meat creates an insulin response, although not as much as dairy, bread, soda, and fake foods.

Of the three primary macronutrients—carbs, protein, and fat—dietary fat is the only one that does not have a significant impact on insulin after a meal. However, eating too much fat could raise insulin over time.

The key to preventing insulin resistance is to maintain extremely low insulin levels periodically. So since we just stated that *all* foods raise insulin to some degree, it makes sense that the only surefire way to keep insulin very low is through the complete voluntary abstinence of food for a set period.

In other words, if you want to keep your insulin levels in check and prevent insulin resistance from destroying your health as it has done to millions of Americans, then fasting must be a regular part of your life. Helping control insulin levels and preventing insulin resistance is just one of the benefits of periodic fasting that we will discuss.

Fasting and Self-Eating

The well-known Gerson cancer therapy advocates fasting extensively. Want to know why? Because when you fast, the body heals. It rests. It finds balance. It gets to do something besides try to digest excess calories.

The process of digestion is taxing and consuming for the human body. In the United States we are always digesting something. We wake up in the morning and start eating—we reach for a bagel or cereal. We eat a midmorning snack, lunch, a midafternoon snack, dinner, and dessert. Then we go to Taco Bell for a late-night "fourth meal."

There are so many issues with overeating, but the most concerning issue with incessant food consumption is that autophagy is never allowed to take place.

Autophagy is a biological process that, on the surface, sounds like science fiction. It is the body's consumption of its own tissue. The term literally means "self-eating." Who knew what was missing in your life was a little self-cannibalism?

Despite how it sounds, autophagy is a good thing.

Even in a healthy human body, cells are continually becoming damaged as a regular part of the metabolic processes. However, as we age and experience stress and free radical damage, our cells become destroyed at an increased rate.

Autophagy then steps in and removes unnecessary or dysfunctional cell components. Think of it as spring cleaning for your internal ecosystem. Damaged cells are eaten away, and newer, healthier cells take their place.

In his book, *Misguided Medicine*, Colin Champ, MD, describes the process as "our body's innate recycling program."[1] Evidence shows that autophagy can help control inflammation and boost immunity. In a 2012 animal study, researchers concluded that autophagy protected against insulin resistance and inflammatory diseases, not to mention cancer, neurodegenerative disorders, and premature signs of aging.[2]

Dr. Champ writes, "Autophagy makes us more efficient machines to get rid of faulty parts, stop cancerous growths, and stop metabolic dysfunction like obesity and diabetes."[3]

Autophagy is so vital that the lack of it can be devastating. One study reported that when mice were prevented from going into autophagy, the results included impaired neurological function, weight gain, lethargy, and high cholesterol.[4]

Autophagy helps to clear damaged cells from the body, including the removal of *senescent cells* that serve no function but still linger inside tissues and organs. The reason it's so important to remove senescent and damaged cells is that they can trigger inflammatory pathways and contribute to the development of various diseases.[5]

When does autophagy occur? Autophagy is active in all cells, but the process increases in response to stress or nutrient deprivation (as in fasting or starvation). This fact means you can utilize "good stressors" such as exercise and temporary calorie restriction (fasting) to boost autophagic processes. Both strategies have been linked to benefits such as weight control and longevity.[6]

How long do you have to fast for autophagy to take place? Studies suggest that fasts between twenty-four and forty-eight hours probably have the most potent effects, but this isn't always doable for many people. You may still receive some of the benefits of autophagy by fasting for a little as twelve to fourteen hours.

An easy way to accomplish this is eating just one or two meals per day rather than grazing on many small meals and snacks. If you usually finish dinner at 6:00 p.m. or 7:00 p.m., try to fast until at least seven o'clock the following morning. Even better, don't eat your first meal of the day until 11:00 a.m. or 12:00 p.m. This is a type of fasting known as intermittent fasting or time-restricted eating that we will discuss in more detail in the next few pages.

To take full advantage of the autophagic process in the body, you might occasionally choose to do a two-day or three-day fast, or potentially longer once you're more experienced with fasting.

If you prefer not to go multiple days without eating, there are options we will discuss.

Another "good stress" that can induce autophagy is exercising. Recent research has shown that "exercise induced autophagy in multiple organs involved in metabolic regulation, such as muscle, liver, pancreas, and adipose tissue."[7]

But is fasting safe for those with certain underlying conditions such as type 2 diabetes, where eating at regular intervals and *not* skipping meals are practices prescribed by medical professionals? It is—with some caveats. But don't let that deter you. We will cover which fasting practices are safest for those with certain conditions in later sections.

The World of Intermittent Fasting

Reaching for food all day long has become programmed into our psyches, and most people do it on autopilot, whether they are hungry or not. When hunger strikes, people clamor to the fast-food drive-throughs and gas stations to fill up on empty calories.

Did you know that once upon a time, eating all day long was associated with being a member of the wealthy, upper class?

Roman emperors are often depicted as fat, lazy sloths who sat around all day while servants stuffed food into their mouths.

In modern times, however, with fast food as cheap as it is (think: Dollar Menu), most socioeconomic classes in America are accustomed to eating from morning until night—and beyond.

In the 1400s, the term *breakfast* was popularized because it describes what is happening when you eat in the morning. You "break the fast." Interestingly, just a hundred years before, the Old English word for dinner was *disner*, and *that* word actually means "to break a fast."

Why? Because dinner after a long day's work was often the first (and only) meal eaten. It wasn't until the late fifteenth century that the term *breakfast* for a morning meal came into use.

Three meals a day (plus snacks) is not the norm for the vast majority of history. Frankly, the accepted practice of eating from sunrise to bedtime is one of the worst-ever crimes against humanity.

We are the *only* mammals on earth that eat all day long.

It's simply not the way we were designed to consume food.

We are the **only** mammals on earth that eat all day long.

Overeating can lead to many things, including obesity and the many lifestyle conditions and diseases associated with being overweight and obese. The solution for regaining control of your appetite, controlling blood sugar, promoting autophagy, allowing your body to heal, and losing weight is *fasting*.

The idea is simple, and right now we are not even talking about restricting the *amount* of food you eat, only *when* you eat it. Scheduling the timing of food intake is known as *intermittent fasting* (often abbreviated as IMF).

Also known as cyclic fasting, IMF is an all-inclusive, general term to describe fasting from food for a few hours a day up to a few days at a time. Most of the fasting methods we will discuss in this book are variations of intermittent fasting.

New science has emerged, showing that intermittent fasting supports a healthy and robust metabolic cycle and protects against obesity and dysmetabolism (more commonly known as metabolic disorder). These benefits significantly reduce your chances of cardiac-related illness.[8] If you can eat in a way that works with your body's natural rhythms, you can work to bring the body back into balance.

Unlike traditional diets that focus on calorie restriction or diets that require you to eliminate certain food groups, intermittent fasting's focus is less on what you eat and requires you to focus on *when* you eat.

It's every dieter's dream—imagine being able to eat without counting calories most days of the week, limiting your intake for one or two days at a time, and still losing weight. Believe it or not, intermittent fasting can make this a reality while also helping to stabilize blood sugar levels, reduce inflammation, and support heart health.

Intermittent fasting's focus is less on what you eat and requires you to focus on *when* you eat.

Typical intermittent fasting times range from fourteen to eighteen hours. The most prolonged IMF period that the most extreme plans would require you to abstain from solid food would be twenty-four to forty-eight hours. In some cases, fasting can last for longer than a few days, but only with careful planning and execution.

We will get into the specifics of how to fast and the best safety practices, but for now, we'll explain it in the most straightforward way possible:

> With intermittent fasting, you abstain from eating for a set period—typically twelve to forty-eight hours. Some intermittent fasting varieties require eating only within set eating "windows," and some plans revolve around restricting calories on some days and eating unrestricted amounts on other days.

There are essential safety precautions that we will address, but intermittent fasting is a simple idea. Notice we didn't say *easy*—but it is an uncomplicated concept.

We are passionate about the benefits of intermittent fasting because they can be life changing. Among other things, fasting may aid with stubborn weight loss, balance hormones, and boost energy and mental focus.

We've seen it work miracles in people's lives in a matter of a few weeks.

We believe that anyone can do it, but it does require a simple mindset shift and a commitment to your health.

In most cases, when you practice intermittent fasting, all you are doing is changing the amount of time during which you eat in a day.

Herschel Walker is a legendary football player and MMA fighter who got quite a bit of media coverage for openly discussing the fact that he's been eating just one meal a day for over twenty years. One meal a day for all of that daily training and physical exertion! He is a 225-pound champion who looks and feels phenomenal.

How can that be possible?

We have both been fasting for years. We haven't looked back once. We have learned that not only is it possible, but it is also addictive in all the right ways! Once you make intermittent fasting a part of your life, you'll wonder how you ever ate for so many hours of every day.

Time-Restricted Eating Basics

Now that we've discussed the universal phrase *intermittent fasting* or IMF, we are going to discuss another term for limiting your caloric intake to one window each day.

We're talking about *time-restricted eating* or TRE. Time-restricted eating is when you regularly eat all your daily calories in a shorter time window (such as noon to 6:00 p.m.) than the standard practice of eating all day.

In short, you wait until a specified time (typically lunch or dinner) to consume calories. For example, if you set a TRE window of eight hours, and you finished dinner the night before at 8:00 p.m., you wouldn't consume any calories until the following day at noon.

Many people go their entire lives eating from the time they wake up until the time they go to sleep. If you start eating when you wake up at 6:00 a.m. (the sugary creamer in your coffee counts as breaking the fast), eat three meals, have a snack or two throughout the day, and then have a midnight snack before bed, that equates to an eighteen-hour eating window, and a six-hour fasting window.

Time-restricted eating requires you to flip that ratio.

If eighteen hours of fasting feels too extreme, that's OK! You can still accomplish a great deal with a sixteen-, fourteen-, or even twelve-hour fasting window to start.

What about breakfast being the "most important meal" of the day? There are fewer and fewer people who believe this to be true anymore, but it's certainly something that the cereal manufacturers hope you continue to believe.

The truth is, in biblical times (and even today in other parts of the world), people ate very little if anything in the morning. Then they had a light lunch and consumed their most substantial meal of the day at dinner.

Yet, for most of our lives, we've been told to do the opposite.

While most initial studies on TRE have been done using animals, humans are believed to respond in much the same ways.[9] It makes sense to researchers, considering daily fasting was practiced unintentionally by our ancestors, who didn't have 24/7 access to food.

Without even knowing about the scientifically proven health benefits of fasting, nearly every religious group throughout history has practiced some sort of variation of fasting rituals.

> Nearly every religious group throughout history has practiced some sort of variation of fasting rituals.

Still not convinced? Think about this: Are you sharp after you've eaten a big meal? What about when you're hungry? Don't you feel more alert when you have that twinge of hunger in your belly? Then ask yourself: "Would I want to face a lion in the wild after he's just eaten, or while he's hungry?"

Whether you are about to participate in an athletic event, a test in school, a business presentation, or a television taping, you are sharper when you haven't eaten, and your body is running on its reserves and excess fat stores.

According to researchers at the Regulatory Biology Laboratory at the Salk Institute for Biological Studies, *when* we eat may be as important—or even more important—than what we eat. The Salk Institute in California has been at the forefront of studying the TRE phenomenon, working to understand the health impacts of fasting and how the body reacts when it's forced to fast for a large portion of the day.

Researchers first stumbled upon this breakthrough in animal studies when mice were allowed to eat whatever they wanted, but only during a set time. The mice on the time-restricted eating plan ate what was considered a "poor diet" that was high in calories, sugar, and fat, yet they still didn't gain the weight that researchers expected.[10]

However, once they had access to the same food any time they wanted, the mice's weight gain doubled *despite eating the same number of calories*. Here are the surprising results:[11]

» A nine-hour window of access to food caused a 26 percent weight gain.

» A fifteen-hour window of access to food caused a 43 percent weight gain.

» A twenty-four–hour window of access to food caused a 65 percent weight gain.

Their stunning conclusion was that periods of regularly fasting for twelve to sixteen hours a day could dramatically and positively impact body weight. Time-restricted feeding caused less weight gain than all-hour access for mice eating a high-fat, high-sugar diet over twelve to twenty-six weeks, and it also led to weight *loss* of up to 12 percent when applied to mice that were already obese.

What does this mean for the diet and weight-loss industry? Some TRE proponents believe you can eat whatever you want and still lose weight by limiting the period in which you consume food. They say this could even be true if you *increase* caloric intake—especially calories from fat, as you do on a keto diet.

We have personally witnessed people consume the same foods in equal amounts during a shorter time window and experience both weight loss and improved health.

However, just because you are within your eating window, this doesn't mean you should eat everything under the sun. There are plenty of diet and fasting programs advertised that claim you can eat anything and everything you want in your eating window.

Be wary of plans that offer this advice.

Recent studies indicate that gorging before sunrise and after sunset seems to negate some of the beneficial effects of fasting.[12]

Intermittent fasting methods that utilize time-restricted eating give you a *little* more freedom to eat what you want, and they often eliminate the need to count calories. However, eating lots of junk and fast food during your window to the point of calorie surplus will nullify some of the benefits of fasting and could make it difficult to break past a weight-loss plateau.

Does this mean you can no longer indulge in your favorite foods? No. Just remember that food is and will always be the best—or worst—medicine.

Types of TRE Fasting Schedules

First, we introduced you to intermittent fasting. Then, we explained a more specific type of intermittent fasting called time-restricted eating or TRE. Now we are going to tell you about more precise ways to practice TRE.

If any of this seems confusing, remember that when you break it down, these plans simply require that you abstain from eating for different amounts of time. The fact that there are so many ways to fast is a tremendous benefit because it means that there is a variety of TRE-style fasting that is right for everyone.

The 16/8 fast

Break your fast at noon
  and eat your last meal at 6:00 p.m.

The 16/8 fast is incredibly popular. It's a type of TRE schedule in which you spend sixteen hours of each day consuming only unsweetened, calorie-free liquids. Then, you use the remaining eight hours to eat all meals and snacks.

Many people eat according to this schedule as a part of their routine, while others only do it for a short period for reasons such as weight loss and blood sugar control. As long as the food timing works for your body and makes you feel great, there is no reason that it can't be used over a more extended period.

Please note that while a window from noon to 6:00 p.m. is most common, you are free to choose another eight-hour window, such as 11:00 a.m. to 5:00 p.m. or 2:00 p.m. to 8:00 p.m., if those work better with your lifestyle and schedule.

The 16/8 fast is common in the health and fitness industry and is the backbone of many popular diets and weight-loss plans. If you adequately hydrate and stay busy, you often don't even notice going without food until lunch. After dinner, success hinges on your ability to remind yourself that late-night snacks are keeping your body from adequately resting and even potentially impeding the repair and healing process your body desperately needs.

The warrior fast

Break your fast at 2:00 p.m.
and eat your last meal at 6:00 p.m.

The warrior is a more narrowed TRE plan in which you eat in a four-hour window during every twenty-four hours to mimic how our primitive ancestors would have eaten after hunting and gathering all day. We suppose it could be called the 20/4 plan since it is the same as the 16/8 fast, except that is has a shorter eating window. Once again, there is no reason to believe that this plan could not work over a more extended period, especially considering that humanity once ate in this manner for many centuries.

The 24-hour fast

Eat dinner and then do not eat again
until dinner the next evening.

This fast is not as nearly as hard as it sounds on the surface. While no one likes the idea of not consuming any food all day long, that is not what this fast requires. When you practice the 24-hour fast, you eat dinner the night before, and then you don't eat again until dinner the following evening. The great thing about this plan is that you are not having to go a whole waking day without eating. Instead, you go to bed feeling satisfied and not at all deprived.

This fast can make you feel so great and energized that you may just be tempted to do it again the next day. Just make sure to listen to your body and never push yourself past feelings of extreme dizziness or lethargy.

The alternate-day fast (eat-stop-eat)

Fast one day,
*   eat regularly the next. Repeat.*

This fast requires you to abstain from food every other day, but on your non-fast days, you may choose to consume whatever you want with no restrictions. Some people prefer to use the 24-hour fasting technique for their fasting days so that they don't have to go an entire waking day without food.

This method of fasting is also sometimes called the "eat-stop-eat" method, where you eat nothing from dinner one day until dinner the next day, and on the other days, you eat as you usually would.

Others prefer not to eat anything on their fasting day, effectively making their fasting window last from dinner the night before (6:00 p.m.) until breakfast on the day after their fast (6:00 a.m.). In this instance, you would be utilizing a thirty-six–hour fasting window.

Many people we know (ourselves included) opt to eat clean, organic foods and limit their intake of junk and fake foods on their non-fast days in order to accelerate their results and gain additional health benefits. People choose to eat this way from two days to thirty days and beyond. This fast is a relatively easy one to maintain due to the no-restriction days.

The modified alternate-day fast

*Eat five hundred calories or less one day,
eat regularly the next. Repeat.*

This fast is like the alternate-day fast, except that on your fast days, you may consume up to five hundred calories. Many feel that this style of alternate-day fasting is more realistic to maintain. Some people prefer to drink only liquid on their "fast days" such as fresh vegetable juices and bone broth. We will discuss juice and bone broth cleanses and their innumerable benefits later in this book.

The 5:2 fast

*Choose two days a week to fast
and eat well the other five.*

Finally, the 5:2 fast is a type of TRE when you eat normally for five days a week, and then on the remaining two days that week, you either fast entirely or significantly reduce caloric intake. The days you choose to fast may vary depending on your schedule and preferences. For example, some may choose to fast on Mondays and Fridays, while others may choose Tuesdays and Thursdays as the days when they will abstain from consuming calories.

The Power of a Water Fast

Now that we've discussed the most popular forms of TRE, let's talk about a type of TRE-style fasting that has a reputation for being the toughest and most physically taxing fast.

Of course, we are talking about a water-only fast—the same one that Jesus Himself carried out in the Bible for an astonishing forty days. A water-only plan is the strictest form of fasting we would ever recommend, and it's not meant for everyone without talking to a trusted health professional first.

One of the great fasting pioneers of modern times, naturopathic doctor Paul Bragg, is famous in the fasting world for his recommendation to perform a fast or cleanse two or more days a week. That equates to fifty to one hundred days a year of fasting!

You are not alone in thinking that sounds extreme—but if Bragg's life isn't a testament to the power of fasting, then we don't know what is.

Like many of the other health heroes of his time, such as Jack LaLanne, Bragg began his quest to help others heal after becoming very sick himself. He developed tuberculosis when he was just sixteen years old, and rather than use traditional medical treatments, he developed an eating, breathing, and exercising program.

Among Paul Bragg's healing techniques that included deep breathing, eating organic foods, drinking distilled water, juicing, exercising, and listening to body cues, he also advocated water fasting as one method of promoting longevity. Using these tools, he restructured his body into an ageless, pain-free pillar of health.

A water-only fast is self-explanatory. You consume nothing other than water for a set period. Remember, it may sound intimidating to eat and drink nothing other than water for, say, twenty-four hours, but if you practice the 24-hour fast the way we previously discussed (dinner to dinner), it's far more doable.

Even single-day water fasts can work wonders in your body. Yes, it could be challenging, but the rewards are great. Among other numerous advantages, water fasting has the potential to:

» Reduce blood pressure

» Help shed stubborn pounds

» Improve cell recycling

» Slow down premature aging caused by oxidative damage and inflammation

If you are motivated to unlock the healer from within and wish to reap the many benefits of a water fast, then it's as simple as starting by eating dinner tonight, drinking water during the next twenty-four hours, and then eating dinner the following night.

A quick note that water fasting is not the same as *dry fasting*. Compared to water fasting, dry fasting is much more restrictive. While water fasts permit the consumption of water (and sometimes other beverages such as unsweetened coffee and tea) during the fasting window, a dry fast requires you to restrict *all* foods and drinks, including water.

While some claim that the dry fasting results are much more profound, there's limited evidence to support this. For example, one review published twenty-five articles and found that both types offered similar benefits in terms of weight loss and overall health.[13] Water fasting is also much more flexible and easier to follow. It is also associated with fewer adverse side effects.

If you properly prepare for your fasting periods and have spoken with a trusted health practitioner or coach, there is no reason why you can't safely fast in this manner for a week, two weeks, or longer.

Could you do that? Don't underestimate yourself or your ability to exercise control over your fleshly cravings.

The Daniel Fast

There is one hero in the Bible who recognized the benefits of denying the yearnings of his taste buds and finding strength in the power of the whole, fresh foods, and his God.

Through Daniel's story God gives us a fasting plan that is designed to heal from within and provide restoration, joy, hope, and strength.

The Daniel Fast or Daniel Diet is based upon the prophet Daniel's dietary and spiritual experiences, as recorded in the Book of Daniel. It's a type of partial fast that focuses heavily on vegetables and other whole foods but leaves out any animal-derived food sources. You also abstain from all alcohol and fatty, processed foods during the Daniel Fast.

Then, for a set period, such as ten days, twenty-one days, or even forty days, you eat only clean foods as described in Leviticus 11. There are two references in particular in the Bible that lay the foundation for the diet:

Please test your servants for ten days, and let them give us vegetables [pulses] to eat and water to drink (Daniel 1:12).

In those days, I, Daniel, was mourning three full weeks. I ate no pleasant food, no meat or wine came into my mouth, nor did I anoint myself at all, till three whole weeks were fulfilled (Daniel 10:2–3).

Daniel and his friends, Hananiah, Mishael, and Azariah (more commonly known to us as Shadrach, Meshach, and Abed-Nego), were carted off against their will to Babylon, along with all of Judah's livestock and the temple treasure.

The young men may have been held captive, but that did not stop them from standing up for their health and demanding to live a better way. Daniel and his friends requested to defy orders and follow their eating plan for ten days. Daniel 1:15–16 (NIV) says this about their results:

At the end of the ten days they looked healthier and better nourished than any of the young men who ate the royal food. So the guard took away their choice food and the wine they were to drink and gave them vegetables instead.

Those were the results after just ten days! Can you imagine how much more significant benefits you could gain from eating this way for extended periods?

Whenever we've done the Daniel fast ourselves, the first thing that we always notice is how easily we lose weight, even when that is not the goal. On the fast, you don't count calories, and you can eat as much of the approved foods as you want.

That is why, if you are overweight or obese, the Daniel Fast could be your secret weapon for removing weight quickly and safely and without feeling like you are "starving" yourself. You are free to eat raw fruits, raw vegetables, raw nuts, and raw seeds. You can eat chia, coconut products, and avocado. There are so many amazing foods that are still allowed—and quite frankly, you'll be amazed at the results.

We have devoted a special section at the end of this book to the Daniel Fast for those who want to learn more details, including the spiritual benefits of fasting.

Getting the Most Out of Time-Restricted Eating

Time-restricted eating is quite different from standard "diet" approaches, which usually fall into one of two categories: calorie-restrictive or food-restrictive. Time-restricted eating, on the other hand, allows you to select the foods that work best for you and eat them in any window that you choose.

Fasting for roughly fifteen or sixteen hours a day—or as little as twelve hours—appears to have significant effects on hormone levels that determine your metabolism, blood sugar, and whether you burn fat or sugar as fuel.[14]

The idea that calories may not matter as much as we once believed goes against everything we thought we knew about losing

> # Calories may not matter as much as we once believed.

and gaining weight. However, this is what results from several clinical trials using animals suggest.

Recent eye-opening studies show that by eating during a shortened window each day, your body is more likely to burn fat and keep your weight at a healthy level.[15] This finding seems to be the case without the need to cut calories, avoid entire food groups, or count macronutrients such as carbs and fat.

Maybe it's easy to believe that TRE can work for weight loss, but you wonder if fasting is healthy overall. In the next chapter we will discuss the benefits of fasting in-depth, but here is a partial list of the benefits of practicing time-restricted eating:

» Lower levels of inflammation

» Improved blood sugar levels

» Enhanced detoxification

» More control over appetite hormones

» Enriched heart health

» Better immune response

» Improved brain function

» Faster muscle recovery

If you want to practice some variation of TRE, it's as simple as picking a period during which you will eat, and when you are

> Most of the diseases and conditions we face today are born out of dietary excess.

outside that window, consume only calorie-free drinks such as water, herbal tea, and black coffee.

Most of the diseases and conditions we face today are born out of dietary excess. It makes sense, then, that the solution for finding healing, healthy weight, and vitality is also based on nutritional choices.

PART 3

THE WHY BEHIND FASTING

The Twelve Biggest Benefits of Fasting

Activate the Healer Within

Imagine being able to kick-start your metabolism, feel more energy, and enjoy a variety of health benefits without having to count calories or adhere to strict meal plans.

Say hello to just some of the benefits of fasting.

What makes fasting seem so unusual is that, with all the diet advice out there, the most straightforward and most useful plan might be to simply not eat for a longer stretch of the day than previously thought ideal. Of course, as we discussed earlier, fasting isn't the same as starving yourself.

But fasting isn't a diet, either.

The literal definition of *fasting* is to abstain from food and drink for a specific period—but in this context, we prefer looking at fasting as simply a change in eating patterns.

In place of three meals a day or a handful of frequent smaller meals, you are going to select a specific window of time to eat, whether it's a few set hours a day or particular days of the week. During that time, you can eat food without counting calories and even occasionally indulge in some of your favorite treats.

However, we hate to rain on anyone's parade, but if you continue to eat processed foods and potato chips regularly, it's unlikely you'll reap the full benefits of fasting. If that's you, we encourage you to examine your diet and expand your taste to include whole, fresh foods before trying a fast.

If you practice fasting and also consume a mostly whole-food diet that is rich in fruits, veggies, lean proteins, healthy fats, and raw dairy, you *will* see tangible changes. Then, those occasional splurges on chocolate, cheese, or dinner out won't have as big of an impact as they might if you were on a calorie-restrictive diet.

The beauty of fasting is that there isn't one "correct" way to do it. Multiple types are popular, and they are popular because they work. Remember this: There isn't a single food or supplement that heals you. Turmeric alone doesn't heal you. Ginger doesn't heal you. Fish oil and probiotics don't heal you. Spinach and kale don't either.

> The beauty of fasting is that there isn't one "correct" way to do it.

Your body heals itself.

Fasting works by taking digestion off the body's to-do list, allowing it to focus on healing and regeneration. When you do that, your body starts to produce something called stem cells. Stem cells create new and healthy tissue in your body, helping you heal.

So, if you're looking to overcome digestive issues, seeking to address neurological problems, fighting cancer, trying to lose weight, or many other healthy, worthwhile pursuits, fasting is one of the absolute best things you can do for your body.

Over the next few pages, we are going to highlight the top twelve benefits of fasting. There are more benefits than the ones we discuss here, but these seem to be the most universally sought-after goals and the ones that bring about the most significant transformation, vitality, and healing.

To date, there have already been hundreds of human clinical trials and animal studies that conclusively point to the fact that intermittent fasting can lead to improvements in every major area of health. The practice can also positively influence the battle against conditions such as obesity, cancer, diabetes, cardiovascular disease, and neurological disorders.

Fasting works by taking digestion off the body's to-do list, allowing it to focus on healing and regeneration.

If you are still unsure about fasting, that is understandable. Just stick with us and keep reading. The more you learn about this incredible health tool, the more ready you will be to implement it into your routine.

#1 Lose Weight Quickly

According to the Centers for Disease Control and Prevention (CDC), almost 72 percent of Americans age twenty and older are overweight, a percentage that includes the 40 percent of Americans who are obese.[1]

That means that right now more than 230 million people in this country weigh more than they should. And almost half of those people weigh *significantly* more than they should.

That's a lot of people.

In light of this, is it any wonder why the weight-loss industry hit a new peak in 2018, growing 4 percent to reach $72 billion?[2]

Our fellow Americans are desperate to lose weight, and they are willing to give a lot of money to anyone who promises they have the answers. And bonus points if the solution means that they don't have to change anything about their current lifestyle!

Again, we don't like being the bearers of bad news, but weight-loss magic bullets don't exist. However, if we were to pick one tool that is as about as close to a weight-loss magic bullet as it gets, it would be intermittent fasting.

Dramatic weight loss is possible, and it doesn't have to take nearly as long as we used to think. The idea that the only way to lose weight is to lose one to two pounds a week is contradicted by the results we've seen thousands of people experience through intermittent fasting.

There have been studies that support fasting as a tool for efficient weight loss. One 2015 study found that alternate-day fasting trimmed body weight by up to 7 percent. Whole-day fasting led to similar results, but with up to a 9 percent reduction in body weight.[3]

Another study that examined a 16:8 TRE style of intermittent fasting showed that it successfully reduced fat mass while retaining both strength and muscle mass.[4] This fact is one of the reasons why we recommend the 16:8 fast so often.

Another study out of the University of Southern California placed 71 adults on a five-day partial fast (eating between 750 and 1,100 calories a day) once every three months. Those test subjects lost an average of six pounds, reduced inflammation, shrunk their waistlines, and lost total body fat *without* sacrificing muscle mass.[5]

Fasting helps you lose weight more efficiently by forcing your body to use up fat stores as fuel. When you eat a standard diet, your body uses glucose (sugar) as its primary source of energy and stores whatever is left over as glycogen in your muscles and liver. When you don't give your body a steady stream of glucose all day long, it begins breaking down the glycogen to use as fuel.

Fasting helps you lose weight more efficiently by forcing your body to use up fat stores as fuel.

After the glycogen has been depleted, your body seeks out alternative sources of energy, such as fat cells, which are then broken down to help power your body.

This idea is what drives the popularity of the keto diet, in which you abstain from carbohydrate intake almost entirely to "force" your body to use up stored fat for energy.

If you want to lose weight and lose belly fat, fasting (even irregularly) could be the key. Many people prefer intermittent fasting to traditional diets because it eliminates the need to meticulously measure foods and track the calories and grams consumed.

A study conducted by the University of California San Diego that analyzed 2,200 overweight women found that TRE also has positive effects on immunity and blood sugar control, which are both tied to weight gain.[6] As you also probably know, poor blood sugar control is a risk factor for obesity, type 2 diabetes, and cancer, among other things.

When someone is overly sensitive to insulin, the "fat-storage hormone" that signals cells to take in calories from food, the pancreas produces more, and this promotes the growth of cells, even mutated cancer cells.

After comparing women not eating or drinking anything for at least twelve hours with those who fasted for less than twelve hours, researchers found that women who fasted longer had better blood sugar control than those who didn't fast as long. This result was independent of other eating behaviors, such as how many calories the women were eating.

We would like to note that when you go into a fast with weight loss as the primary goal, you may end up disappointed. While many people lose weight quickly, others experience more gradual results and may even encounter a few weight-loss plateaus here and there.

Fasting improves energy and sleep quality. Fasting promotes healing from within.

That is why we invite you to put your focus on the other benefits you will gain from a fast and less on the number on your scale.

Fasting improves energy and sleep quality. Fasting promotes healing from within. So keep that bigger picture in mind as we continue to discuss the benefits of fasting.

#2 Detoxify Your Body

Environmental scholars report that earth and its inhabitants are being inundated with man-made chemicals at a rate unlike anything in our history. We're talking about the air we breathe, the water we drink and bathe in, and the food we eat.[7] We are also talking about the chemicals in clothing, in the carpet, in personal care products, cleaning products, new car smell, furniture, and much more.

You name it—it's toxic.

Over the years, so many of us have accumulated high levels of heavy metals. That doesn't even take into consideration all of the pathogens that live inside the body. The good news is fasting is one of the best and quickest ways to eliminate toxins.

> Fasting is one of the best and quickest ways to eliminate toxins.

One of the things we want to make sure you take away from this book is that God designed the body to heal itself. Instead of this mentality, however, the norm in our society is to think, "What pill can I take to feel better?"

The answer is never found in what we take *in to* our bodies because the answer is already there! In many cases, what we need to do is remove the interference and allow our organs to rest so they can work properly.

Think about this: every time you eat fat, for instance, your liver and gallbladder must work to break that down in order to put it to use, get rid of it, or store it for later use. If you don't eat anything for a more extended period than usual (such as sixteen hours or more), your liver now has the opportunity to rid itself of heavy metals and toxins and chemicals.[8]

When you rest your systems, they are better able to detox.

If you have an extremely hectic lifestyle (and really, who doesn't these days?), you are always on the go with too much to do and not enough time to do it. Now imagine if your spouse and children went on a trip without you, and all of a sudden, you find yourself at home alone in pure solitude.

What would you do with all that time?

You may watch a few shows on Netflix, but you also might be inspired to start straightening up around the house. Maybe it's time to clean out the garage and the closet. It seems like the ideal time to clean the whole house from top to bottom.

Your body does the same thing when it's allowed to take a break from the digestive process. When you do not eat or you eat clean, minimal amounts of food, you take the burden off your digestive system, and your body goes into its own "spring cleaning" mode. This idea is also the driving principle behind both acupuncture and chiropractic care: Remove the interference and let the body heal.

When you rest your systems, they are better able to detox.

#3 Sharpen Your Mind

If you are about to go into a big presentation, what is probably the last thing on your mind? We would guess that you are not thinking about eating a big, heavy meal.

The reason is that we are naturally more alert when we are hungrier. There is a reason why everyone naps after Thanksgiving dinner. Big meals make us sleepy! It's also the reason why you feel like taking an afternoon siesta at work after an enormous lunch.

Large amounts of food are not ideal when you want to be your most alert.

If you have issues with mental clarity and focus, fasting and cleansing can uncloud your thinking and help sharpen your mind like nothing we've seen.

Like involuntary starvation, voluntary fasting is viewed by your body as a stressor. However, it is a *positive stressor* that is temporarily taxing on the body but still incredibly beneficial.

Positive stressors are essential because they cause the body to adapt in ways that promote health and fight disease—and one of the ways it adapts during a fasting period is to hone mental sharpness and alertness.

Fasting has also been shown to have anti-aging effects on the brain by helping to improve neuroplasticity, which is the brain's ability to form new neural connections. Fasting can also help fight inflammation, and a decrease in inflammation has been linked to improved memory.

One animal study showed that intermittent fasting helps enhance cognitive function and protect against changes in memory

Fasting is a *positive stressor* that is temporarily taxing on the body but still incredibly beneficial.

and learning function compared to a control group.[9] Another animal study found that intermittent fasting protects the brains of mice by influencing specific proteins involved in brain aging.[10]

Additionally, the anti-inflammatory effects of intermittent fasting may also help slow the progression of neurodegenerative disorders such as Alzheimer's disease.[11]

Fasting is shown to help with mood enhancement, which could be great news for your coworkers and family if you are prone to mood swings. There is a reason why every holistic clinic, natural health retreat, ancient medicine practitioner, and even some modern medical establishments use fasting and cleansing as a part of their cognitive therapies. It works!

#4 Decrease Chronic Inflammation

Acute inflammation (such as swelling at the site of an injury) is a normal part of the immune process. Slow, festering, chronic inflammation, on the other hand, can lead to chronic disease. Some research has even linked inflammation to conditions such as heart disease, type 2 diabetes, obesity, and cancer.

When you do a fast or a cleanse, you could dramatically reduce chronic systemic inflammation. This benefit has been demonstrated through some fascinating research on the near-complete cessation of rheumatoid arthritis pain after a period of intermittent fasting.[12]

Fasting has also long been used to reduce inflammation and protect against cell damage. Studies show that fasting can suppress the expression of inflammatory markers and decrease oxidative stress.[13] One study conducted in Florida, for example, found that alternate-day fasting was able to reduce levels of oxidative stress after just three weeks.[14]

A study published in *Nutrition Research* examined 50 adults observing Ramadan and reported that they had decreased levels of some inflammatory markers during Ramadan fasting.[15] Another 2015 study found that a longer duration of fasting was associated with a decrease in inflammation markers.[16] In the journal *Rejuvenation Research*, alternate-day fasting helped reduce markers of oxidative stress.[17]

While more research is needed, these studies provide promising evidence showing that IMF may help reduce inflammation and fight off chronic disease.

If fasting helps reduce inflammation, promote detoxification, and reduce cravings, it is natural to assume that diseases preceded by these risk factors will be less likely. For example, there is research to support the fact that longer duration fasting cycles may help slow the growth of tumors.[18] Another study reported that intermittent fasting effectively suppressed the production of pro-inflammatory immune cells, leading to decreased inflammation in the body.[19]

We always say that it is far less expensive and less painful to prevent cancer and other diseases than it is to treat them. Fasting is not a guarantee that you will never develop a deadly disease. Still, considering the role it plays in decreasing chronic inflammation (and the fact that it's free to utilize), it is certainly worth trying.

#5 Reduce Cravings

We have some excellent news for the hungriest among us.

Fasting can normalize ghrelin levels.

Ghrelin is known as the hunger hormone because it is responsible for signaling to your body that it time to eat through the feeling of hunger. Serial dieting and restrictive eating can increase ghrelin production, which will leave you feeling hungrier. But when you fast, though you might find it challenging for the first few days, you will help normalize ghrelin levels over time.[20]

Eventually, you won't feel hungry simply because it's your usual mealtime and your body is used to eating then. Instead, your body will become more adept at discerning when it actually *needs* food.

Leptin, also known as the satiety hormone, is produced by the fat cells that helps signal when it's time to stop eating. Your leptin levels drop when you're hungry and increase when you're feeling full.

Because leptin is produced in the fat cells, those who are overweight or obese tend to have higher amounts of leptin circulating in the body. Too much leptin floating around can cause leptin resistance, which makes it harder for the body to turn off hunger cues effectively. Leptin resistance then leads to overeating and the inability to stop eating when full.

One study measured leptin levels during intermittent fasting and found the level to be lower at night during the fasting period.[21] Lower levels of leptin could translate to reduced leptin resistance, reduced hunger, and potentially even more weight loss.

#6 Slow the Aging Process

While not yet conclusively proven in humans, animal studies link intermittent fasting with increased longevity. One study found that intermittent fasting increased life span in rodents.[22] Another found that a group of mice who fasted intermittently lived longer than the control group, even though they were heavier than the non-fasting mice.[23] It's not a given that the same results would occur in humans, but the results are encouraging.

Fasting could be about as close to a "fountain of youth" as we can get. Studies show that it improves both your physical appearance and complexion. We saw this clearly with Daniel and his friends in the Bible. After only ten days, the difference in their appearance and the other healthy young men was noticeable to everyone!

Fasting could be about as close to a "fountain of youth" as we can get.

After a few weeks of fasting, don't be surprised to hear people say, "Wow, you look great!" They may even wonder if you've been to a spa for a facial. It may motivate you to take a before picture of your face and then another one after ten to fourteen days of IMF. The results won't lie.

#7 Normalize Insulin and Blood Sugar

When you consistently and habitually take in excess carbs and sugar, the body tends to become insulin resistant, which could pave the way for a host of chronic diseases, including type 2 diabetes.

When you eat, carbohydrates are broken down into glucose (sugar) in your bloodstream. A hormone called insulin is responsible for transporting the glucose out of the blood and into the cells where it can be used up as energy. Insulin doesn't work as effectively when you have diabetes. This dysfunction can result in high blood sugar levels, coupled with symptoms such as fatigue, thirst, and frequent urination.

If you don't want to go down this path, it's critical to keep your body sensitive to insulin. Some studies have found that intermittent fasting benefits your blood sugar levels by keeping them well-regulated and preventing spikes and crashes.

A study published in the *World Journal of Diabetes* found that intermittent fasting in adults with type 2 diabetes improved key markers for those individuals, including their body weight and glucose levels.[24] Another study found that intermittent fasting was as effective as caloric restriction in reducing visceral fat mass and insulin resistance.[25]

In yet another study, participants with diabetes fasted up to sixteen hours daily for two weeks. Not only did intermittent fasting cause weight loss and a decrease in caloric intake, but it also helped significantly reduce blood sugar levels.[26]

If you're struggling with prediabetes or insulin sensitivity, intermittent fasting can get your numbers going in the right direction again.

#8 Promote Heart Health

One of the most impressive intermittent fasting benefits is its favorable effect on heart health. Studies show that intermittent fasting improves your heart health by lowering certain heart disease risk factors.

When you consume too much of the bad (LDL) cholesterol, your triglyceride levels increase, which then increases your risk of heart disease. Intermittent fasting can help lower LDL cholesterol levels, decreasing triglycerides in the process.[27]

Another interesting thing to note is that fasting doesn't appear to adversely affect the levels of good (HDL) cholesterol in the body. In one study, fasting was shown to increase good HDL cholesterol and decreased both LDL cholesterol and triglyceride levels.[28]

In another study published in the *Journal of Nutritional Biochemistry*, intermittent fasting was shown to cause an increase in levels of adiponectin.[29] Adiponectin is a protein involved in the metabolism of fat and sugar that may be protective against heart disease and heart attacks.[30]

#9 Help Break Addictions

Addiction to junk food is one of the most commonly cited reasons people give us for not being able to fast. Ironically, fasting has been shown to help break addictions to processed foods, but that means that there may be a period when you have to overcome the urge to stop at your favorite fast-food drive-through with your desire to be well and feel good again.

As kids, our big treats in life were often food-based—footlong hotdogs, pizza nights, birthday cake, and more. We are conditioned from a young age to equate food with pleasure and relaxation. When we become adults, we face other addictions, such as gambling, pornography, video games, drugs, and alcohol.

We are addicted to many things, and one of those is undoubtedly food. We use it to "medicate" us when we are stressed, bored, and tired. The good news is fasting can help *break* that addiction and other addictions as well.

When you fast, your willpower will be restored, and you will feel empowered like you may not have felt in years. Edward Earle Purinton, who wrote a book called *The Philosophy of Fasting*, had this to say, "There is not a habit or weakness that can survive a siege of prayer and fasting. Prayer alone is just one half of the battle."[31]

Those of you who pray, you've got a double portion of success coming. Do you have something in your life that's coming against you? Take siege and take it by force, with prayer, and with fasting.

#10 Reduce Stress and Improve Sleep

One of the more surprising benefits of fasting is that it helps reduce stress and promotes better sleep.

Fasting helps reduce stress and promotes better sleep.

Fasting can't reduce or remove the *sources* of your stress. The circumstances that may bring pressure and anxiety into your life may still be there. However, fasting can help calm your body's stress responses and make you better able to cope with specific situations. The primary way fasting accomplishes this is by lowering your cortisol levels, the chemical that signals the fight or flight response in your body.

Practicing fasting also improves your body's ability to deal with stress at a cellular level. Intermittent fasting activates cellular stress response pathways similar to very mild stressors, acting as slight stimulants for your body's stress response. As this occurs consistently, your body is slowly reinforced against cellular stress and is then less susceptible to cellular aging and disease development.[32]

Surprisingly to some, fasting can also help you sleep better. This country suffers under the tremendous weight of a collective sleep crisis. People don't often talk about it openly, but we are not sleeping enough, which is a significant problem considering sleep is our body's time of restoration and rebuilding.

You will sleep better when you unburden your body through fasting.

#11 Heal the Gut

One of our favorite things about fasting is what it can do for your digestive tract. When you fast, you allow your gut to rest.

Dr. Oda H. F. Birchinger, who supervised more than seventy thousand fasts as a pastor in Texas, had this to say, "Fasting is a royal road to healing, for anyone who agrees to take it, for recovery and regeneration of the body, mind, and spirit."[33]

The road to healing for many originates in the gut. As Hippocrates once said, "All disease begins in the gut."[34] Scientists have since discovered that most of your immune system (some estimate as much as 70 percent) resides in your digestive tract, so it needs to be in the best shape possible.[35]

The digestive tract is the area of your body that is most exposed to environmental threats, including bacteria, viruses, parasites, and toxins.

When food is broken down in the gut, it travels through the blood to the liver, the largest organ of the body's natural detoxification system. The liver breaks down and removes the toxic byproducts produced by digestion, including both the natural ones and the poisonous chemicals present in our modern food supply.

During a fast, organs such as the liver are given a break from the hard work of digesting foods. They are now free to detoxify! The extra energy and lessened workload provide the body a chance to restore itself, while the burning of stored calories helps get rid of stored toxic substances.

When you fast, you allow your gut to rest.

#12 Balance Your Hormones

Finally, let's talk about hormones, the body's chemical messengers.

Fasting has been shown in particular to improve female hormonal balance, helping lessen the severity of PMS and symptoms of menopause such as hot flashes.[36]

Fasting also promotes the secretion of human growth hormone. Human growth hormone, or HGH, is naturally produced by the body, but only remains active in the bloodstream for a few minutes. HGH has been effectively used to treat obesity and help build muscle mass, which is essential for burning fat and slowing the aging process.[37] HGH also helps increase muscle strength, which can improve your workouts.

Intermittent fasting optimizes the body's HGH levels in two ways. First, it keeps insulin levels low for the majority of the day (the length of your fasting window).[38] Research indicates that insulin spikes tend to disrupt the natural production of HGH. Second, it can help decrease body fat,[39] which also directly affects HGH production. There have been numerous other studies that showed dramatic increases in HGH production after just a few days of fasting.[40]

It is important to note that fasting can also negatively impact hormones if it is done improperly or done by individuals in specific risk categories. Women have the potential to be more impacted by these effects than men.[41]

Fasting isn't meant to become a source of stress, but in some people with compromised or high cortisol and adrenaline levels, a further increase in these hormones from fasting can result in some unwanted side effects.

If you have existing adrenal or hormonal issues or you tried TRE but noticed excessive fatigue, anxiety, and irregular periods due to hormone disruption, time-restricted eating might not be right for you. Alternatively, you may need to try a more modified fasting style. For more on this and how to ease into fasting, refer to the FAQs later in the book.

God's creative power within your body can heal.

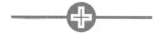

We believe that God created you to heal and to regenerate. God didn't make a mistake when He created your body—and just because you are sick today does not mean you must remain unhealthy for the rest of your life.

When you break your arm, do you expect that bone to heal? Then why can't that happen to other parts of your body, including an organ or an entire body system that may be suffering from dysfunction?

God's creative power within your body can heal.

If you have fallen into the trap of believing the lie that as we age, we must naturally feel a little bit worse day after day, we invite you to journey into the realm of possibility and give fasting a try.

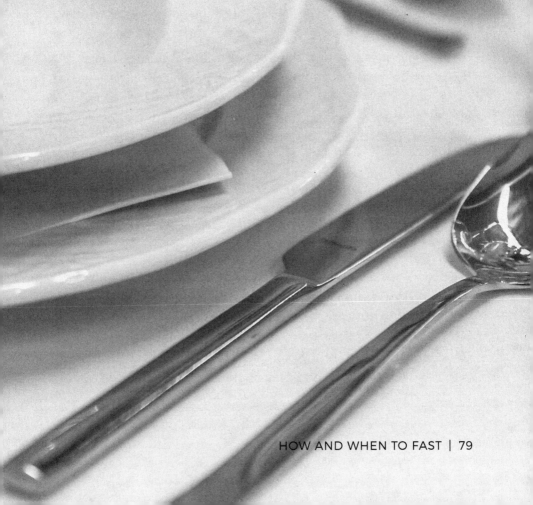

PART 4

HOW AND WHEN TO FAST

Fasting and Eating Strategies

There Is No One-Size-Fits-All Fasting

We've learned a lot so far.

By now you know the most common variations of time-restricted eating. You've learned about the Daniel Fast, and you might have even asked yourself whether you could ever do a water-only fast.

You also know that fasting is anything but a modern fad, and you read about the most significant, most impactful benefits of fasting. Now it's time to address something you may be thinking: "What exactly are these guys going to ask me to do?"

It's a fair question, and the answer is straightforward. First, the goals are to help you regain control of your body, lose weight, increase insulin sensitivity, help you sleep better and think more clearly, and encourage the body's natural healing processes. You will accomplish that and more by doing two main things:

1. Find a sustainable way to make fasting a more regular part of your life.

2. Make better food choices during your daily eating window.

Perhaps just as important, let's talk about something we are *not* going to do. We are not going to put a trendy label on this. There are benefits to the popular diet plans—and we have recommended programs such as keto, Paleo, Whole30, Mediterranean, Okinawa, GAPS, and Dukan to many people. However, the beauty of fasting is that no matter what food philosophy or dietary plan you adhere to, fasting works in them all.

Each diet or eating style has certain benefits associated with it. The problem with fad diet plans is the games they play with our psyches because they are all rooted in one word: *restriction*.

As much as it may not look like it on the surface, fasting is actually about opening you up to the *world of possibility* when it comes to healing, balance, and restoration.

> Fasting is actually about opening you up to the ***world of possibility*** when it comes to healing, balance, and restoration.

Restrictive plans are not sustainable for many people and could have unexpected, negative repercussions. Carb-elimination diets are hard to get right. If you go keto but are not doing daily breath or blood analysis to test ketone levels and practicing carb cycling to protect your gut biome, you may not see the results you want.

Let's forget about labels for a moment and focus on foods that will cause the desired physiological changes to your internal ecosystem, which include organic vegetables, clean proteins, and healing fats. Then you can gain even more benefits when you affect your physiology by adjusting your food intake to a specific window of time every day.

The goal is to find a daily feeding window that leaves you energized and satiated without the need for starchy carbs or sugars.

Fasting can bring tremendous health and blessings into your life, but if it's done incorrectly, it can also be detrimental. So you want to fast in the right way. For example, if you are fasting to lose weight, but you feel weak and dizzy the entire time, and you gain all of the weight back within a week or two, you have not done your body any favors. You may have also done tremendous damage to your psyche and your confidence in fasting.

In our experience, fasting will produce the best results when done periodically, not permanently. Are there some people (like Hershel Walker, who we mentioned earlier in the book) who practice IMF for years on end? Sure. But we are all different, with different needs and vastly different tolerance levels.

Fasting will produce the best results when done periodically, not permanently.

All of this simply means that there are no one-size-fits-all fasting regimens we can give you that work for everyone. You have to become your body's number-one advocate by listening to it and adjusting your plans, even if they worked perfectly for someone else.

In this chapter, we are going to cover how to fast safely and effectively. However, before we can get to that, we feel it's critical first to discuss how to approach eating.

There will always be both in your life: periods of eating and periods of fasting. They are both necessary and both significant. If you fast but do not eat well, you may still see some results from fasting. However, poor eating habits quickly catch up with you during times when you are not practicing time-restricted eating.

So it's essential to make good food choices that sustain and bring life into your body, whether you are in a period of fasting or not.

Learn to Shift Your Focus

When it comes to losing weight and keeping it off, and when it comes to reversing disease, we aren't interested in fads. That said, we think that the modern diet trends such as the Paleo and veggie-rich keto diets are primarily the way we should all be eating. The healthiest versions of these plans advocate a grain-free, processed-dairy-free diet with plenty of veggies, healthy fats, and clean proteins.

In essence, we believe in eating the way humans ate before foods became processed, and modern farming practices poisoned our foods, including our grains.

> The backbone of any healthy, sustainable plan should be a natural style of eating called *intuitive eating*.

We also invite you to take advantage of a few other proven eating strategies. For example, we believe that the backbone of any healthy, sustainable plan should be a natural style of eating called *intuitive eating*.

Staying present in the moment throughout the day, remaining conscious of changes in your body, and practicing intuitive eating will allow you to course-correct and also become aware of food sensitivities.

The *real* epidemic we face in this country—and the reason why fasting is so effective at making you aware of your food choices and hunger levels—is *unconscious eating*. We stuff our faces in the darkness of a movie theater. We go for seconds and thirds at the buffet, with no thought about the amount of food we are putting into our bodies. We binge watch our favorite TV shows while we mindlessly binge on our favorite takeout.

That style of food consumption will not bring health into your life. However, it's also true that there is no universal eating plan that will unquestionably work for everyone. If we've learned one thing after working with thousands of patients over the years, it's that no two bodies are the same.

What works for one person may fail for another, no matter how similar the two may seem. This statement is also true when it comes to fasting. Intermittent fasting works well for some people over more extended periods. For others, practicing IMF for longer than ninety days may start to produce diminishing returns.

Some people find that when they practice IMF but don't take in enough healthy protein, fat, fiber, and nutrient-dense fruits and vegetables during that time, they never feel quite right.

That is why *intuitive eating* is the "secret sauce" that helps optimize your eating and fasting plan according to your unique chemistry.

The **real** epidemic we face in this country is *unconscious eating*.

Fasting isn't a diet.
It's a lifestyle change.

The reason we start diets and then fall off the bandwagon is that they seem so arbitrary, with no rhyme or reason. We have plenty of rhyme and reason for what we are advocating.

Fasting isn't a diet.

It's a lifestyle change.

On the surface, the consumption of food seems straightforward. In its most simplistic form, the proper way to eat and fast could be summarized as follows:

- » Eat real food, mostly raw plants.
- » Eat clean meat that ate real food.
- » Drink fresh, clean water.

Practice fasting fifty to one hundred days a year.

The problem is, many people will easily disregard these simple instructions. The reason rests in psychology, and more specifically, the psychology of eating. The *psychology of eating* refers to how someone's thoughts, emotions, beliefs about their abilities, personal history, and lifestyle habits affect what and how much they eat and their overall biological function. It takes into account more than just what types of food a person chooses to eat and avoid. It addresses other influences on our eating habits such as:

» The *mind-body connection*, which is the impact that someone's mental state has on numerous aspects of his or her overall health (including food choices). Multiple studies have shown that the levels of emotional stress individuals are under have strong ties to both the quality of their diet and to how well they can use the nutrients they obtain from food to maintain a healthy weight.[1]

» Overall *outlook on life*, including how individuals feel about their diet, significantly impacts food choices as well as bodily functions, including digestion, metabolism, sleep, libido, and much more.[2]

» *Body image*, or the way someone feels about his or her own body, weight, and health, can also affect food choices. Poor body image, coupled with a dysfunctional relationship with eating and food, can also contribute to addictions, eating disorders, and yo-yo dieting that can all lead to long-term metabolic damage.[3]

The civilizations of antiquity didn't have the options we have today—they either ate real food or no food. Before grocery stores and restaurants, every bit of nutrition came directly from the ground, the water, or the field. Chemicals were not sprayed onto crops. Livestock was not given genetically manufactured feed. Food was not prepared in hazardous plastic and coated metal containers.

Today, however, it is a different story. It's impossible not to know someone who suffers from food addiction, struggles with overeating or obesity, or is suffering from some preventable disease brought on by a poor diet.

That is why fasting is a great equalizer.

All things remaining the same (your environment, the personal care products you use, etc.), by removing food, you can more easily determine if what you were eating is the cause of your issues.

Once you determine that food is the culprit of a specific issue, you can begin to experiment with removing certain foods altogether to find the precise triggers of your bloating, fatigue, weight gain, and more.

Food Addictions Are Real

Our relationship with food is complicated. It represents existence itself in the form of life-giving energy and nutrition. Still, it also carries with it the potency of being a *natural reward* that we all look forward to at various points in the day.

Like anything else that brings pleasure, relief, or enjoyment to human beings (alcohol, illicit drugs, gambling, sex, etc.), food can be addictive.[4] Remember, sin came into this world because Eve could not resist tasting the forbidden fruit.

Perhaps because dieting has become so commonplace—and both good and bad food choices abound—food addictions are generally less accepted than other types of addictions, contributing to what some experts call "fat stigma."[5]

Fat stigma and fat phobia are growing phenomena in our culture that are turning even a discussion of food addiction into a taboo subject. *Fat phobia* is a fear or dislike of extremely overweight and obese people. *Fat stigma* is an attitude that could manifest in different ways. It may exhibit as a disapproving glare from a stranger at an obese individual, a person who moves when an overweight person sits down next to him or her, or an employer who loses interest the moment someone who is overweight walks in for a job interview.

The bottom line is many people who are not overweight look at those who are with antipathy and think things like, "Why don't they just work out?" or "Can't they just stop eating so much?"

Yet, for anyone who has ever dealt with a food addiction, they know the solution is never that simple.

Food is a drug, which is "a medicine or other substance which has a physiological effect when ingested or otherwise introduced into the body."[6] You can probably recall a time when eating your favorite food was the highlight of your day. People with food addictions desire those feelings in the same way that a person addicted to any other drug feels after taking his or her drug of choice.[7]

Several specific triggers and causes have been identified that seem to be directly linked to the further development of food addictions:

1. *Food as a reward*—dopamine is considered a critical *reward chemical* that is activated in pleasure centers of the brain in response to eating delicious foods. High levels of dopamine release can be linked with the intake of certain calorie-dense foods, provoking someone to enjoy repeatedly eating the food in order to experience those positive feelings.[8]

2. *Emotional eating*—study findings show that regular emotional eating (eating for psychological reasons rather than because of physical hunger) contributes to the development of food addictions. Emotional eating creates a vicious cycle since the act leads to altered moods, and those altered moods can lead to damaging food choices. For example, sadness can lead to cravings for more sugar.[9]

3. *Serial dieting*—another common trigger that leads to addictions is a long history of serial dieting. In many cases, people can engage in both categories of dysfunctional eating (calorie restriction and food addiction) at different stages in their life. A history of dieting and calorie restriction increases the odds of overeating, developing a food addiction, and gaining weight in the future.[10]

The following tips will provide you with several possible actions and helpful ideas for dealing with food addictions and their consequences:

» **Consider seeking professional help.** A professional can serve as a coach, keep you accountable, and help you recognize the connections between your emotions and eating habits.

» **Practice the 80/20 rule.** Try not to view foods in terms of which ones are "good" or "bad." Instead, focus on how different foods make you feel and if they supply you with the nutrients and energy you need. Give yourself a break 20 percent of the time and eat a little more freely, allowing you to stay focused on eating well the other 80 percent of the time. Fasting makes this a little bit easier, as studies show that indulging from time to time when you are following a TRE-style eating plan is less damaging than when you eat all day long.[11]

» **Learn mindful eating.** Practicing mindful eating involves becoming highly aware of your habits, preferences, and triggers. It also means approaching weight loss from a place of better body acceptance and a goal of becoming healthier, rather than just aiming to become thinner or "more attractive."

» **Focus on nutrient density.** When you are within your eating window, make an effort to crowd out less healthy foods by focusing on the positive: filling your plate with real, whole foods of all colors and varieties. Try to avoid processed foods that trigger you into overeating and feeling out of control. The more processed foods you consume in your eating window, the harder it will be to stick to your intermittent fasting schedule at all, as those food addictions will come calling, and you may not be able to resist.

» **Find new passions and hobbies.** Incorporate more healthy hobbies into your life that take your mind off fasting and eating, such as volunteering, hiking, cycling, gardening, joining fitness groups at your local gym, painting, etc.

» **Pick your influences wisely.** It's been said that you become the average of the five people with whom you surround yourself with the most. Write down the people in your life who are negative, discouraging, and regularly steer you away from healthy eating habits. Then write down five people in your life who are encouraging, healthy, and have a positive influence. Those are the people with whom you should be spending your time.

When you practice these in conjunction with some intermittent fasting, the results may astound you. However, it is also important to note that while fasting is a great tool, in some people with a history of eating disorders, fasting can trigger unhealthy behaviors from the past.[12] It's essential to acknowledge and address these issues before you try a fast.

Programmed to Eat

According to John S, Allen, Ph.D., author of *The Omnivorous Mind*, all humans have a "theory" that guides how, how much, and what we eat. These *food theories* start to take shape in childhood under familial and cultural influences and then continue to develop throughout adulthood based on many societal, cultural, economic, and technological factors.[13]

The training our minds undergo regarding food and eating habits is intricate, but it is also an innate, natural function. Newborns less than a minute old seek out their mother's milk. Our stomachs grumble, signaling that it's time to refuel. For most, eating seems as natural as breathing and requires little thought for many years.

However, if your diet needs to change for health reasons or you want to incorporate fasting into your routine, your cognitive theories about food intake will suddenly need to be examined and adjusted.

Unfortunately, once that programming is set in our minds, it is no easy task to rewrite. The mind is not comfortable with new theories about food and wants to go back to what is familiar. This is one of the reasons people backslide on their diets, engage in yo-yo dieting, and find it nearly impossible to skip a meal or two.

So we are going to examine two popular food theories that are designed to help guide food choices more naturally. For both, we will discuss the basics behind the theory, what foods make the cut, and some of the reasons for choosing that style of eating.

Keep in mind that for it to work, be sustainable, and offer the most benefits, a theory has to fit your lifestyle, preferences, and values.

While it's not essential to adhere to a well-defined food theory to be healthy and maintain ideal nutrition—nor is it necessary to comply with one defined approach to benefit from intermittent fasting—there are some advantages associated with following a food theory:

» Food theories can offer a way to bond with others as they are commonly tied to cultural and family traditions.

» Food theories can be beneficial when managing an existing health condition.

» Some people follow specific food theories to take the guesswork out of what to eat.

» Others adhere to a theory because of its benefits for the environment, such as choosing to eat local, organic, and sustainably produced food.

In the context of fasting, we strongly feel that following a food theory may make fasting more approachable and feasible. So read with an open mind and consider which ideas resonate most with you and your personality and priorities.

CLEAN EATING

Striving to eat nothing but whole, non-denatured food that is ideally organic, locally grown, and sustainably raised.

Clean eating is all about consuming whole foods that are as close to nature as possible. Preferably, you want to eat foods that have not been overprocessed and are organic, locally grown, and sustainably raised. Some people who are clean eaters are also proponents of raw foods over prepared, cooked meals.

Today conventionally grown vegetables and animal foods are deficient in nutrients and loaded with pesticides, which must be processed by the immune system and may lead to chronic disease.

The Environmental Working Group created a yearly updated list of the most and least contaminated foods based on 43,000 sample tests for pesticide residues on produce collected by the US Department of Agriculture and the Food and Drug Administration.[14] When it comes to eating clean, many who follow this food theory feel more comfortable opting for a conventionally grown fruit or veggie from the Clean Fifteen list. However, if you genuinely want to eat clean, all produce consumed from the Dirty Dozen list must be organic.[15]

The Dirty Dozen

1. Strawberries	7. Peaches
2. Spinach	8. Cherries
3. Kale	9. Pears
4. Nectarines	10. Tomatoes
5. Apples	11. Celery
6. Grapes	12. Potatoes

The Clean Fifteen

1. Avocados	9. Cauliflower
2. Sweet corn	10. Cantaloupe
3. Pineapple	11. Broccoli
4. Onions	12. Mushrooms
5. Papaya	13. Cabbage
6. Sweet peas (frozen)	14. Honeydew melon
7. Eggplants	15. Kiwifruit
8. Asparagus	

It's also vital that your animal proteins be as clean as possible. Most of the time, this means the meat is organic (which also means the animals ate organic meals), free-range, grass-fed, or wild-caught. Eating clean just makes sense for people who want to eliminate processed, inflammation-causing fake foods from their diets and reduce their chances of developing lifestyle-related diseases such as type 2 diabetes and heart disease.

SATIETY EATING

A focus on slow, deliberate eating so that you eat until satisfied but not beyond, to only consume the number of calories that your body requires.

According to Merriam-Webster, satiety means "the quality or state of being fed or gratified to or beyond capacity."[16] Satiety is a critical element of most diet plans, as it has to do with learning about the body's subtle signals related to fullness and hunger. Research suggests that several ways to help eat up to the point of comfortable satiety include:

- » Eating slowly
- » Sitting down to eat
- » Thoroughly chewing food
- » Eating similar foods over and over again
- » Choosing unprocessed foods
- » Enjoying a variety of foods within one meal
- » Using smaller dishes to help psychologically

The *chewing theory* to reach satiety is based on the idea that about thirty-five chews per mouthful of food will help to slow down the meal and prevent weight gain by alerting the person early on in the meal as to when it's best to stop eating.

A study conducted at Oxford Brookes University compared thirty-five chews with ten chews per mouthful to test this theory. Researchers found that higher chewing counts reduced food intake despite increasing chewing speed, and despite doubling meal duration before participants claimed to feel "comfortably full."[17]

There are no real risks associated with attempting to eat until reaching satiety, although it may be difficult at first to master. Mostly everyone will, at times, eat more than the precise amount they need to feel comfortably full. Occasionally eating past satiety isn't a problem unless it happens frequently and becomes an ingrained habit.

There are plenty of other food theories not discussed here. We did not address the raw food theory, the 90/10 Theory (where you eat clean 90 percent of the time), the DNA diet, and vegetarian and vegan lifestyles.

There is no universal food theory or diet that works for everyone. You must pick the elements that work for you and combine them to create a healthy plan, and perhaps more importantly, sustainable for your lifestyle.

We've discussed how to eat, and so now it's time to talk about how to "not eat." You'd think it'd be as simple as "just stop eating," but there are a few considerations and a few simple steps to take that ensure a higher degree of success.

How to Fast Safely

Intermittent fasting should be viewed as a change in lifestyle rather than a diet. Unlike diets, with fasting, there's no need to count points or calories or plug your foods into a food diary after each meal.

Still, to reap the most benefits possible, focus on filling your plate with healthy whole foods during the days that you eat to fill up on nutrients rather than empty calories.

Additionally, always listen to your body. If you feel weakness or fatigue when you go an entire day with no food, try increasing your intake a bit and have a light meal or snack. Alternatively, try out one of the other methods of intermittent fasting and find what works for you.

Ready to try a fast? Follow these steps for a more effective and rewarding experience.

1. DECIDE WHAT TYPE OF FAST YOU'RE GOING TO DO.

If you are new to fasting, we recommend easing in with time re stricted eating, starting with twelve hours of fasting. If that feels good after a few days, you can increase the fast to fourteen hours and up to eighteen. For the majority of people, we do not recommend fasting for longer than that if you plan to make it a regular practice.

The ideal goal for most fasters is to utilize the 16:8 method. If you don't eat anything between 8:00 p.m. and 12:00 p.m. the next day, for instance, you've already fasted for sixteen hours. Typically, carrying out this plan involves skipping your evening snack after dinner and then skipping breakfast the next morning.

Have you fasted before? Then you might want to try a more ambitious fast such as alternate day fasting. Or maybe you are ready for a water-only fast.

If you are struggling with a particular issue such as hypertension and would like to prevent it from developing into something more serious such as type 2 diabetes, a more extended period fasting could be one of the greatest things you can do for your body.

A more extended fasting period may also be appropriate for those doing a spiritual cleansing (more on that later in the book). Just be sure to pay close attention to the safety issues and contra-indications in part five.

2. SET SOME GOALS AND CONSIDER TELLING OTHERS.

What do you want to accomplish by fasting? Do you want to lose weight, be healthier, feel better, or have more energy? Whatever your goals are, you should write them down and place them where you'll frequently see them during your fast.

Let's use weight loss as an example. While it's a great goal, it shouldn't be your only goal. What if you wake up for three days in a row and don't see any change in the scale, but you feel less bloated, you are sleeping through the night, and you have ten times more energy during the day? These are huge wins and must not be discounted by focusing purely on the scale.

After you write down your goal, you may choose to tell other people about it. However, don't skip the "writing it down" step, because telling people is not enough. According to recent research, telling friends and family about what you want to achieve creates a premature sense of completeness.[18] It may make you feel a temporary sense of pride in deciding to do a good thing, but that pride may not be enough to motivate you when the going gets tough.[19]

On the other hand, writing down your intentions and reviewing them creates a gap between where you are and where you want to be—and your brain feels compelled to find a way to close that gap.[20] Telling other people about your plans without actively reminding your brain, "Hey, we're not there yet, and we need to keep striving toward this goal" will artificially close that gap in your mind.

The mental aspect of fasting and, truthfully, making *any* lifestyle change is complicated. The best thing you can do is be honest with yourself and become more aware of your self-talk. Keep the words you say to yourself (even the ones that never come out) as positive as possible.

3. EASE INTO ALL-DAY AND MULTIPLE-DAY FASTS.

When you are new to intermittent fasting, it may be best to add it to your routine just once or twice a week, and on nonconsecutive days. Don't be too hard on yourself if it takes you a few weeks or even a few months to break the habit of continuously eating.

One thing you want to avoid is feeling stressed or anxious because you are fasting. This response can have adverse effects on your health. Remember, you are not a hero or a warrior by going from gorging yourself one day to fasting the next. There are safe ways and reckless ways to prepare for a fast.

4. PLAN AHEAD AND BE PREPARED.

The day before

The day before a fast is not a day to binge eat. Don't use it as an excuse to eat cake or an entire pizza. It's also a good idea to avoid eating excessive amounts of salty, sugary foods as they spark cravings and the desire to snack more. Remember that alcohol can be dehydrating, so consider not consuming any alcohol just before or during a fast.

Timing

You can technically schedule your fasting window for any twelve-to sixteen-hour block you choose. We recommend starting it two to three hours before bed, and then extending it for at least another two to three hours after you wake up each morning.

The potential problem with choosing to eat as soon as you wake up (especially if you're an early riser) is that you will need to stop eating reasonably early in the day. Going to bed hungry will make it more difficult to fall asleep and get the rest you need. If you are new to fasting, trying to go from 7:00 or 8:00 p.m. to 9:00 or 10:00 a.m. the next day and increase from there.

Food planning

Before beginning your fast, decide when you're eating and *what* you'll be eating. Knowing this in advance takes off some of the pressure. You don't want to have to make decisions about what to eat while you are fasting. If you do that, you may decide to eat whatever is most convenient because you are so hungry.

We have a variety of recipes at the end of this book that will give you good ideas for what to eat when you are not fasting. We include breakfast foods, main dishes, soups, smoothies, and more. There is always a delicious, healthy option if you take the time to plan.

As you become more used to fasting, you might find it's unnecessary to sort out meals beforehand, but having a range of healthy food waiting makes fasting a lot easier.

Hydration

One of the keys to a good fast is to stay hydrated and avoid dehydrating foods. Experts recommend eating plenty of clean protein, healthy fats, and fibrous foods. There is no reason to remove carbs before a fast unless you are on a keto diet. Carbs can help keep your energy levels up during the fast.

A note about coffee

If you plan to do a fast without caffeine and are a big coffee or tea drinker, plan to start tapering your intake one week before your fast to avoid caffeine withdrawal and side effects such as headaches and nausea. Even those who drink one cup per day could benefit from a reduction in caffeine a few days before their fast.

While these ideas will help you feel better during your fast, there is nothing you can do, drink, or eat the day before that will prevent you from feeling hungry while fasting. Overeating may have the opposite effect and make you more hungry than usual the next day.

Your body deserves a little understanding and some grace as it sheds old habits and learns new ones. Listen to your body!

5. LISTEN TO YOUR BODY.

It can take some time to acclimate to the new feelings you may experience during fasting. It can also take some time to get used to your new eating schedule. That is why it's essential not to be too hard on yourself if you try for a sixteen-hour fasting window and only make it twelve hours.

Your body deserves a little understanding and some grace as it sheds old habits and learns new ones. Listen to your body! If you are in hour ten of a sixteen-hour fast and feel like you need a snack, then have one. If your fasting time is technically over, but you're not hungry yet, wait until you are.

Cut Yourself Some Slack

There are no hard and fast rules here.

You're not "messing up" if your plan changes.

You might find it helpful to jot down a sentence or two each day about how you felt during your fasting window. You may also find that certain times of the month or year, different types of fasts work better.

When you are fasting, resist the urge to count calories. Make your fasting time the focus of the plan. If you have been practicing intermittent fasting for some time and are still not seeing results, it may be time to look at caloric consumption or what foods you may need to reduce or eliminate.

When you do eat, consume mindfully. Don't sit down and eat as though you've never had a meal before. That's where food planning comes in handy. Do your best to stick to lean meats, organic raw dairy, and quality carbs such as ancient grains, fruits, and veggies. These are all components of what we call a healing diet (see a fuller list of healing diet–approved foods in the appendix).

Fortunately, the research suggests that you don't need to follow a time-restricted eating schedule every single day to see results. Eating within an eight- or nine-hour window most days of the week can be highly beneficial. Dave Zinczenko, the author of the bestselling book, *The 8-Hour Diet*, recommends following time-restricted eating just three or four days a week.[21]

More research is still needed to determine the ideal meal schedule and fasting period. But honestly, we feel that a universal eating window—one that works for every single person—does not exist. We are all diverse, with unique needs and a myriad of other factors that make what is "ideal" look very different.

You are your number-one advocate. Don't forget that, and also don't forget that God gave you a body that is designed to heal itself. You are indeed fearfully and wonderfully made!

PART 5

FASTING FAQS

Troubleshooting and Common Issues

Identifying Roadblocks before They Appear

The first question we often hear when we talk about fasting is, "How hard could it be? Don't I just stop eating?"

As you are now beginning to understand, while it is *that* straightforward, it's not quite *that* simple. If you want to achieve long-term success, there is some planning and goal setting required, and there are also some safety considerations, especially for certain groups of people. In the next few pages we will cover those safety considerations and answer the most commonly asked questions that arise during fasting.

Fasting is one of the powerful spiritual breakthrough tools.

Purposefully abstaining from food for a period has been a practice carried out for thousands of years by people around the world. Ancient fasters once turned to fasting primarily for spiritual or religious reasons. We still believe fasting is one of the most power-ful spiritual breakthrough tools as well. We also know that a large body of research indicates that fasting may also be one of the most effective ways to not only lose weight but also to help improve health markers and even improve your overall quality of life.

Intermittent fasting is by far the most popular type of fasting, thanks in large part to the fact that it takes advantage of sleep time and only requires, in most cases, that you forego an evening snack and then skip breakfast the following day. Of course, that is not the only way to do an intermittent fast, but it's undoubtedly the easiest way for newcomers to dip their toe in the water and see how they feel.

The remainder of this chapter will focus on troubleshooting the most common fasting issues and solutions for them. We hope that as you continue in your fasting journey, you will keep this book on hand as a reference guide when you run into a stumbling block or other questions while fasting. The best issues to encounter are the ones you were already expecting!

AM I SUPPOSED TO FEEL SLUGGISH WHILE FASTING?

Fasting can unquestionably improve overall health, but there are also some precautions that everyone should take into consider-ation. Perhaps the most commonly cited reason we hear for people abandoning a fast is they felt "off" or unusually tired and sluggish.

If you start to feel sluggish or dizzy at any time, it may be wise to eat something. While you can expect to feel hunger during a fast, dizziness (particularly during a typical daily TRE-style fast when you are not going an entire day with no food) is a sign that there is an imbalance that you need to address.

If you've ever tried fasting but felt sluggish or moody, you were likely making one or more of the most common fasting mistakes that we will cover in this chapter. These missteps include not correctly hydrating, eating too much or too little, fasting too much too soon, or trying to engage in strenuous exercise while fasting. We will cover all of those and more in the pages that follow.

AM I DEHYDRATED OR LACKING ELECTROLYTES?

A portion of the fluids we take in throughout the day come from water-dense foods such as fruits and vegetables. We obtain approximately 20 percent of our daily water intake from food! So when you're not eating, you must drink more fluids than usual to avoid dehydration.

During your fasting window, we recommend sipping on hydrating beverages between meals—liquids such as water, herbal tea, or bone broth. Drinking enough water may help ease hunger pangs and is beneficial for other critical bodily processes, such as digestion and detoxification.

Meanwhile, bone broth is considered one of the best ways to stay hydrated *and* replenish key electrolytes, such as calcium, magnesium, and other trace minerals that are depleted throughout the day. While bone broth does contain a small number of calories, we still recommend drinking a cup or two throughout the day, especially if you are feeling a little sluggish (more on bone broth cleanses in the final section of this book).

Experts recommend that even on non-fasting days, adults should drink half of their body weight in ounces. That means if you weigh 160 pounds, you should be drinking at least eighty ounces of water every single day. This recommendation is a minimum, and for most people, we suggest consuming as much as a gallon of water a day during a fast. It sounds like a lot—but sipping on water all day long is a great way to lessen hunger pangs and stay energized.

PRO TIP: SUPER-HYDRATE

One smart way to ensure you are taking in enough water is to "super-hydrate" first thing in the morning. Put a large glass of water by your bed (thirty-two ounces is a good target) and drink that first thing upon rising. It will quell any extreme hunger pangs and give your body a jolt of energy. Plus, you'll already be well on your way to reaching your daily intake target.

AM I EATING THE *WRONG* FOODS?

The reason intermittent fasting is doable for so many people is the fact that you're not giving up food for days on end. By simply extending the amount of time between dinner and breakfast or skipping breakfast or dinner, you can reap incredible benefits.

That said, when you are within your eating window, it's best to stay away from unhealthy, processed foods. Since you're eating less frequently while fasting, it's even more important to make sure you get all the essential nutrients that you require when you do eat.

Filling up on lots of empty calories from foods such as refined grains, unhealthy fats, and sugary snacks will likely result in you taking in lower levels of certain nutrients—especially vital electrolytes and essential vitamins. To get the most out of fasting and ensure that you feel your best during the process, we recommend adopting a healing diet that consists of lots of organic produce, healthy fats, and high-quality lean protein. Eating clean foods will also help

To get the most out of fasting and ensure that you feel your best during the process, adopt a healing diet that consists of lots of organic produce, healthy fats, and high-quality lean protein.

prevent symptoms such as fatigue, muscle spasms, weakness, and brain fog. (For a quick and easy reference guide on foods recommended in a healing diet and the foods to avoid, please refer to the appendix.)

AM I EATING *ENOUGH* FOOD?

Nutrient deficiencies are even more likely if you're under-eating during your intermittent fast—particularly if you're active, which further increases your nutrient and energy needs. Additionally, hunger pangs can make it challenging to work or sleep if you're not eating enough.

Women, especially, should be careful not to under-eat or restrict calories too much while fasting. When you are within your eating window, do not deprive yourself and eat until satisfied. Studies regarding intermittent fasting for women show that undereating can harm reproductive hormones, menstruation, and emotional well-being.[1]

We cannot overemphasize that intermittent fasting could cause hormonal imbalance and other unintended and unhealthy consequences in women if it's not done correctly.[2] Women's bodies are more susceptible to signals of starvation. If your body perceives that it is starving, it will ramp up its production of the hunger hormones leptin and ghrelin.

So when women experience insatiable hunger after under-eating, they are experiencing the increased production of these hormones. It's the female body's way of protecting a potential fetus—even when a woman is not pregnant.

Of course, though, many women ignore these hunger cues, causing the signals to get even louder. Or, worse, they try to ignore them, then fail and binge later, then follow that up with under-eating and starvation again. And guess what? That vicious cycle can throw your hormones out of whack and even halt ovulation.

In animal studies, after two weeks of intermittent fasting, female rats stopped having menstrual cycles, and their ovaries shrunk while experiencing more insomnia than their male counterparts (though the male rats did experience lower testosterone production).[3]

Unfortunately, we have yet to see many human studies that explore the differences between intermittent fasting for men and women. Still, the animal studies confirm our suspicion: intermittent fasting for long periods can sometimes throw off a woman's hormonal balance, cause fertility problems, and exacerbate eating disorders such as anorexia, bulimia, and binge eating.

To avoid these consequences, we recommend adding more calories to meals via healthy fats such as coconut oil and avocado. These fats will help stabilize appetite and blood sugar levels.

PRO TIP: Try Crescendo Fasting

Intermittent fasting for women can be hard on the body if you are new to it or if you jump in too quickly. So if you are a woman or you are trying fasting for the first time, you might benefit from a modified fast known as *crescendo fasting*.

Crescendo fasting requires you to fast only a few days a week instead of every day. In this way, it is similar to the 5:2 fast but then combines that with TRE principles.

Amy Shah, a double board-certified doctor, notes that she has seen women benefit significantly from doing fasting this way without accidentally throwing their hormones into a frenzy. It's an all-around gentler approach that helps the body more easily adapt to fasting. If women do it right, it can be a fantastic way to shave off body fat, improve inflammatory markers, and gain energy.[4]

Not all women need to do crescendo fasting, but it will ensure success if you are on the fence, nervous about fasting, or already have existing hormonal imbalances. Here are the general rules of crescendo fasting:

1. Fast on two to three nonconsecutive days per week (e.g., Tuesday, Thursday, and Saturday).
2. On fasting days, do only yoga or light cardio.
3. Ideally, fast twelve to sixteen hours.
4. Eat normally on your intense exercise days.

5. Drink plenty of water (tea and coffee are OK as long as there is no added milk or sweetener).

6. After two weeks, you may be ready to add one more day of fasting.

7. Consider using a bone broth or collagen protein supplement during your cleansing window. These have minimal calories but provide fuel to muscles and can take the edge off hunger and fatigue.

If you have failed at intermittent fasting before, try the crescendo style for a better, more sustainable experience.

For more information on how to spot a macronutrient (protein, fat, carbs) deficiency in your diet, see the "Macronutrient Deficiency" table in the appendix. We also have a special table in the appendix on food group recommendations based on their micronutrient (vitamin and mineral) content.

AM I FASTING TOO MUCH?

Just like other components of a healthy lifestyle—such as clean eating and exercising—it's easy to fall into the trap of believing that more is always better. But just as overtraining can lead to injury, sleep difficulties, and elevated cortisol levels, fasting too much or too often can also have counterproductive effects.

Most experts recommend fasting from two to four days per week, as any more than this may negatively affect metabolism, performance, and appetite. At some point, your body will think it's in serious trouble and start to defend itself against perceived starvation. It's also important to consider the length of your fasting window while doing an intermittent fast, as too large of a window can result in very high hunger levels that trigger uncontrollable or binge eating.

It can take some trial and error to figure out the fasting frequency that's best for you. Start with one to two fasting days per week, each fasting window lasting about twelve to fourteen hours. Once you're used to this routine, you can then consider adding one additional day of fasting or extending your fasts up to fifteen to eighteen hours if that feels right to your body and makes sense for your routine and lifestyle.

AM I EXERCISING TOO MUCH WHILE FASTING?

Some people may be able to engage in intense workouts on fasting days (especially if they are healthy and accustomed to regular activity). You might even find that when eating on a time-restricted schedule, you feel more energetic in the mornings and wish to workout. On more restrictive fasts, however, your low-calorie days might leave you feeling low on fuel. That is why the majority of fasters will feel better when they allow the body more rest and sleep during fasting days.

Experts recommend skipping intense workouts such as HIIT or long aerobic training sessions on days when you take in less fuel. Instead, gentler, therapeutic exercises such as a walk or yoga are usually a better fit on fasting days. These calmer workouts will help prevent symptoms such as fatigue, dizziness, and weakness. If you're fasting for longer than seventy-two hours, however, it's advisable to limit physical activity.

And no matter what day of the week it is—whether you're fasting or not—remember that getting good sleep is always essential for repairing the body and maintaining healthy digestion, detoxification, and hormonal balance. Aim for at least seven to nine hours per night to prevent cravings, low energy, and moodiness.

WHAT ARE SOME OF THE COMMON SIDE EFFECTS?

We've covered a lot of the issues you may experience during fasting. Now we will cover some side effects that may take some getting used to but are to be expected (and not a sign that you have done something incorrectly or are dealing with an internal imbalance).

"Fuel source" adjustments

Most people in America are "sugar burners." If you aren't sure, ask yourself how quickly you get hungry (or possibly hangry) again after you eat. If you can't go too long between meals, you are a sugar burner.

Fasting helps you become a "fat burner." Fat is the superior fuel source, one that prevents the telltale crash we've all felt after eating a meal that is high in sugar and carbs. Keto dieters know that restricting their carb intake helps their body become an efficient fat burner.

> Fasting helps you become a "fat burner."

Fasting can help with that too!

Here's what that would look like if you measure your glucose levels: When you begin to fast, you will notice a leveling off of glucose levels. Then, when you eat your first meal to break the fast, the macros you eat will determine what happens next.

If you eat carbs, sugar, and processed protein, your insulin is going to climb. If you eat healthy fats and clean foods, your insulin response will be minimal, and your body will continue to use its fat stores for energy (the basic concept that drives the keto diet).

Fasting puts your body into fat-burning mode, where your body uses fat for fuel. As a result, you will see an influx of free fatty acids, but you will not see glucose in your blood. Glucose only enters into the bloodstream as a result of intake—and that's it.

Fat is the only macronutrient that doesn't create an insulin response directly. Even protein will create an insulin spike if you eat large amounts. Your body will produce glucose in response to high protein intake. The process is called *gluconeogenesis*, a response that indirectly stimulates an insulin spike. That is why high amounts of protein are not ideal for those who are type 2 diabetic, prediabetic, or at higher risk of developing type 2 diabetes.

When you put glucose into your system, your body has to do something with it. Too much glucose intake over time causes excess fat stores, and eventually, the body starts to store fat where it shouldn't, in peripheral fat stores. That leads to conditions such as a fatty liver and a fatty pancreas.

The autophagy prompted through fasting can help fix that. Once you allow the body to go into autophagy, you can start to burn the fat system-wide (including the fat in your pancreas and other organs). This process is a significant component in the quest to lose weight and positively impact specific disease markers.[5]

Digestion changes

It is important to note that you will see some digestion and elimination changes, particularly on a water-only fast or liquid-only fast such as a juice cleanse.

One of the main aspects of your fast that will determine how much it changes your digestion is food timing. Our digestive system, like every other system in the body, works best and most efficiently on a regular cycle. We are in full "digest" mode when the sun is up, and then digestion slows down at night. This idea is backed up by research that shows that melatonin (whose production ramps up in the evening to promote sleep) sends signals to the liver to slow its activity.[6]

Therefore, it is best to keep your eating window confined to the daytime and early evening and not extend it into the late evening, as the body will have greater difficulty digesting what you eat after the sun goes down.

Possible flu-like symptoms

There have been some cases of fatigue and even flu-like symptoms that may cause you to say, "This is making me sick" or "This is not worth it."

We know those kinds of feelings can be frustrating and cause you to think about abandoning fasting. However, there is a good chance that if you are feeling this way, you may have pushed a little too hard. If your diet is still primarily made of processed foods, fasting may be harder than it needs to be.

In general, you are more likely to feel achy or even sick (this is sometimes called the "keto flu" in the ketogenic world) if you're new to fasting or have never tried a ketogenic diet before. Another reason you may not feel well is if you consume a large number of carbs and processed foods just before fasting.

Slow and steady wins the race when it comes to fasting.

Slow and steady wins the race when it comes to fasting. It's not a weight-loss contest or a test of will and strength. Start slowly. Fix your diet one meal and one fasting window at a time. Drink a little bone broth if you start to feel unwell. Take care of your body, and it will take care of you.

HOW LONG SHOULD I FAST?

There truly is no set amount of time to fast that is right for everyone. Instead of focusing on how long you should fast, it's better to keep a few things about fasting in mind instead:

» If you're genuinely hungry, eat something. If you don't, you'll spend your time a) hungry, b) stressed about being hungry, and c) hungry and stressed (or even hangry!).

» If you're still in the early stages of making healthier food choices and choosing whole foods, it may be best to wait before beginning a fasting routine. Concentrate on eating whole, good-for-you foods first.

» Are you training for a big event, such as a marathon or triathlon? Now is probably not the right time to try fasting. Speak with your coach and doctor first.

» Listen to your body!

Focus on filling up with lots of water, herbal teas, and bone broth during your fasting window and then focus on filling up with nutrient-rich foods when you eat. Discipline is a crucial component, but you must also give yourself some grace because you will slip up from time to time. You may feel like you need a snack during your fasting window or eat dessert made with real sugar. If you fall off one day, jump back on the next. We aren't judging you!

> Discipline is a crucial component, but you must also give yourself some grace because you will slip up from time to time.

WHAT LIQUIDS CAN I CONSUME?

If you're on a time-restricted fast and you're in your fasting window, it's best to stick to no- or low-calorie drinks such as water, coffee and tea (with no creamer or sugar).

Some people enjoy a little bit of stevia in their tea or coffee. As long as stevia agrees with your belly, go for it. Stevia, a natural sweetener with no calories, has surprisingly been shown to have a positive effect on blood sugar levels. In a study on mice, when rodents were fed a high-fat diet over a long period, they eventually developed diabetes. However, this does not seem to be the case for mice who also received a daily dose of stevioside—one of the active components of stevia extract. The mice given the stevia were more protected against diabetes and saw fewer cases.[7]

If you're on an alternate day diet or the 5:2 fast, even during low-calorie hours, you can technically drink whatever you'd like— but remember liquid calories still count. Would you rather spend one hundred calories on a crunchy, sweet apple or a glass of milk? It's your call.

We also recommend abstaining from alcohol during fasting. Obviously, given the caloric density of alcohol, you should not consume it during your fasting window. Drinking it during your eating times may not derail your efforts. However, we recommend not drinking your calories but eating them through nutritious foods, smoothies, and soups. It is important to note that experts have correlated moderate to heavy drinking with weight gain and obesity in humans.[8]

HOW DO I BREAK THE FAST?

Once you have fasted, the "hard work" is over! But that doesn't mean you can start eating everything you want again right away, particularly in the case of fasts that last twenty-four hours or longer. You'll want to be especially mindful of the foods you choose to eat for that first post-fast meal. Post-fast meal selection is vital if you're going to get the maximum benefits from the fast and also avoid feeling sluggish or getting intestinal distress.

The good news is that a review in the *New England Journal of Medicine* reported that fasting periods activate cell pathways that fortify your defenses against stress and illness. When you break the fast and begin to eat again, your cells switch into a state of adaptability. This on/off switch that takes place thanks to fasting is highly beneficial for your metabolic health.[9]

However, depending on the length of your fast (particularly if the fast is water-only and lasts for more than twenty-four hours), the protective mucus lining of your stomach may have been temporarily diminished, which makes the stomach walls more vulnerable to irritation. With this in mind, it's wise not to break your fast with foods or beverages that could irritate the stomach lining, such as coffee, spicy foods, and dairy.

Instead, focus on foods that are easier to digest and gentler on your stomach. We generally recommend a little bone broth to ease your way out of a fast. If you are vegan, you may choose to sip on some vegetable broth or simply eat some raw fruit. In general, here is a list of foods that are acceptable and gentle enough to eat just after a longer cleanse or water-only fast:

» Raw fruit: watermelon, grapes, and apples are fruits that you can easily digest and assimilate.

- » Broth: bone broth and vegetable broth nourish the gut and make you feel satisfied.
- » Cooked and raw veggies and soups: organic vegetable juices and vegetables are ideal foods for after a fast.
- » Well-cooked grains, beans, and pulses: pulses (the edible seeds of plants in the legume family) and grains are the most difficult for the body to break down. So make sure to eat them only when the stomach's lining has enough time to cushion.

When you reach the end of your fasting window, the goal should be to consume a blood sugar–balancing meal that includes protein, fat, and fiber. One example of such a meal would be some wild-caught fish (around four ounces), half an avocado, and about two cups of cooked leafy greens.

Additionally, the probiotics in fermented veggies or a tablespoon of apple cider vinegar about fifteen minutes before you eat can help your digestion get back up and running smoothly.

And don't forget the water! It may feel like all you want to do is eat, but hydration continues to remain at the top of the priority list. Additionally, if you have done a more prolonged fast, you will need to replenish your body with some much-needed electrolytes. You can achieve this by adding a pinch of Himalayan sea salt along with a squeeze of lemon to your fish and veggies.

For more information on how to spot a macronutrient (protein, fat, carbs) deficiency in your diet, see the "Macronutrient Deficiency" table in the appendix. We also have a special table in the appendix on food group recommendations based on their micronutrient (vitamin and mineral) content.

WHAT IF I'M DIABETIC?

TRE might not be for everyone, and some people appear to do better with practicing various types of fasting in general than others. Fasting has an undeniable impact on blood sugar, so anyone dealing with low blood sugar (hypoglycemia) should steer clear of fasting until glucose and insulin levels are well managed.

If you are insulin-dependent, fasting must be a well-monitored endeavor to avoid a hypoglycemic event. You cannot fast and continue to take insulin in large amounts without checking your blood sugar. With no sugar for the insulin to drive out, you will experience a hypoglycemic state.

If you start feeling the telltale signs of hypoglycemia, the eventual goal will be to stop reaching for juice or candy. Sugar packets, candy bars, and fruit juice are not the answer to sating blood sugar lows. If that's how you "treated" blood sugar lows in the past, now is the time to retrain yourself to reach for a piece of low-glycemic fruit instead.

Think about the flawed paradigm under which type 2 diabetes operates. Doctors, in general, assume that people with diabetes have no control over their physiology, insulin production, or even their ability to control food cravings. So they have to be "managed" with medication. If patients take too much of the medication, their blood sugar drops, and they are then expected to compensate by putting sugar in the system, as opposed to not taking as much medication.

Don't look to what you can put *in* to get your blood sugar back up; look to what's causing your blood sugar to go down in the first place. Stop taking so much insulin. You will notice a marked decrease in the amount of insulin you need when you start eating whole foods and fasting. Waning dependence on insulin is a good indicator that you're moving in the right direction. While we have seen many type 2 diabetics successfully reduce and, in some cases, even remove the need for insulin supplementation, you should always consult with a qualified medical professional to discuss the safest ways to go about this.

Insulin is not something you need unless you need it. In other words, if the body doesn't require it to break down all the sugar you are ingesting, why take it?

You must listen to your body.

You must also test—and remember that this book is not a substitute for speaking with your health practitioner about intermittent fasting if you are currently on medication for type 2 diabetes or other conditions.

WHO SHOULD TAKE EXTRA PRECAUTIONS WHEN FASTING?

Fasting is a powerful tool, but it's not a tool designed for everyone. Taking a purposeful break from food is a type of stress on your body. There are ideal times to fast, and there are other times when you should avoid it altogether. And remember, it's best to check with your doctor before beginning a fast. Functional medicine professionals and health coaches may also be able to recommend the type of fast that is right for your specific needs based on your medical history and goals.

The following groups of people should exercise caution and take extra steps in picking the right fast:

1. If you suffer from low blood sugar

If you are hypoglycemic, going without eating all day may lead to dangerous drops in blood sugar. Such drops could cause some unpleasant symptoms such as shakiness, heart palpitations, and fatigue. Start slowly and increase your fasting window with patience and caution. Don't be ashamed to sip on some bone broth during your fasting window.

2. If you have diabetes

As we covered earlier, fasting is a worthwhile endeavor for type 2 diabetics. But, while fasting is probably a healthy pursuit for you, check with a health practitioner before and let them know that you are planning to start intermittent fasting.

3. If you have cancer

This book is not intended as a treatment or substitute for any formal treatment. That said, fasting is a phenomenal tool to use, along with many others in the quest to beat cancer. One study reported that patients who fasted during their chemotherapy treatments reported a reduction in fatigue, weakness, and gastrointestinal side effects.[10] From these results, it's safe to say that fasting is a safe way to alleviate some of the side effects of cancer treatments. We have personally seen fasting bring great healing into the lives of friends and family who have beaten cancer.

WHO SHOULD AVOID FASTING ALTOGETHER?

There are seven groups of individuals for whom fasting is not the right choice for various reasons. If you find yourself in one or more of these categories, you should avoid fasting:

1. If you are an adolescent

Children and teenagers who are still growing should not practice intermittent fasting. Intermittent fasting has not been studied enough in children to assess its safety, so it's best to steer clear while you are in periods of growth.

2. If you are pregnant

Those who are pregnant should also avoid intermittent fasting and focus instead on eating a nutritious diet rich in vitamins and minerals. It is also not advisable to fast while breastfeeding, as long periods of fasting may adversely affect milk production.

3. If you have a history of eating disorders

If you have a history of anorexia or bulimia or otherwise struggle with other psychological eating disorders, fasting could exacerbate those problems. An eating disorder is one condition with which you absolutely should *not* do fasting. Instead, always work with your doctor when struggling with any sort of disorder.

4. If you have gallstone disease

Fasting may increase the risk of gallbladder problems. When you fast, your gallbladder doesn't release bile. As your liver continues to deliver bile, it becomes concentrated. Breaking your fast means your gallbladder could forcefully release sludge or small stones from that buildup that could get stuck in the bile duct. If you have gallbladder issues, proceed cautiously with intermittent fasting. A study published in the *American Journal of Public Health* stated that people with gallstone disease reported increased hospitalization risk after fasting.[11]

5. If you have adrenal fatigue

Fasting could elevate cortisol, stressing your already-overworked adrenals. In one study, a group of healthy females fasted for forty-eight hours and displayed elevated cortisol levels throughout the fast.[12] The "good stress" may just be too much on your adrenals if you have adrenal fatigue, or if your adrenals are already overworked from chronic stress.

6. If you have thyroid issues

Your thyroid performs many functions, including balancing energy, body temperature, and emotions. According to studies, fasting can cause "profound changes" in the function in the hypothalamus-pituitary-thyroid (HPT) axis.[13] Another study found that short-term intermittent-style fasting and more extended fasting periods both resulted in up to a 50 percent decrease in active T3 hormone.[14] This decrease is not ideal as it may result in a worsening hypothyroid condition.

7. If you are sick

Your body typically needs a steady supply of nutrients when you are feeling under the weather. Although the adage "starve a fever" is well known for a reason, it is not advisable to go entirely without any nourishment when you are sick. Instead, focus on taking in foods and supplements that supplement the immune system, such as bone broths, fresh vegetable juices, nutrient-dense protein shakes, and green drinks with added turmeric and ginger. The last thing you want to add to your plate when you are sick is the stress (albeit a beneficial form of stress in healthy people) caused by fasting.

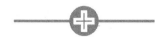

You already have everything inside you that it takes to break through limitations, plateaus, and roadblocks. We encourage you to take your fasting journey one day at a time. Have dinner the night before at 6:00 p.m. and don't have a snack before bed. Then wait until 8:00 a.m. to 10:00 a.m. the next morning to eat breakfast. And bam! You've already fasted for twelve to fourteen hours!

With so many types of intermittent fasting plans to choose from, you can find one that fits your lifestyle. Intermittent fasting is not a good fit for everyone, especially those suffering from certain health conditions. However, for many people it is an excellent addition to an otherwise healthy lifestyle.

You can do this.

PART 6

SMART FASTING TOOLS

Supplements, Supporting
Practices, and Cleanses

When Fasting Needs a Helping Hand

If you are ready to give fasting a try, you now know everything you need to know to make it happen.

While we both believe that food and fasting are the *best* and most effective "medicine" we have at our disposal, we also know that there are specific supplements and practices that can support and even enhance your fasting efforts.

In this final chapter, you will learn about which essential oils most greatly benefit your body during a fast and beyond. We will also briefly discuss the use of ketones, a supplement used frequently by fasting and keto diet enthusiasts.

Additionally, we'll talk about the importance of self-care, goal setting, and motivation before we end this chapter by highlighting a few additional ways to modify fasting to fit your unique needs and goals. These include a juice cleanse and bone broth cleanse.

As a bonus, we have also included a unique, must-read final section on the spiritual benefits of fasting. If you tried fasting before and failed, we encourage you to look within and find a reason for fasting that transcends how you physically look and feel.

Fasting and Essential Oils

Fasting boasts significant benefits for your weight, your mood, and your sleep, and every system in your body. When you combine fasting with the right type of essential oils, it can amplify the overall benefits. There are five essential oils we recommend to those who are planning to practice intermittent fasting.

> When you combine fasting with the right type of essential oils, it can amplify the overall benefits.

FRANKINCENSE OIL

Often called the "king of oils," frankincense is powerful, effective, and incredibly therapeutic. For thousands of years, religious followers have used frankincense during worship, meditation, and spiritual practices. The word *frankincense* appears seventeen times in the Bible, and the word *incense* is mentioned 113 times; in such cases, incense is often assumed to imply frankincense along with myrrh and other spices.

Frankincense has extraordinary health benefits. It is used to help relieve chronic stress and anxiety, reduce pain and inflammation, boost immunity, and even combat tumors. The terpenes in frankincense enable it to go beyond the blood-brain barrier.[1] It also increases the activity of leukocytes, which help the body fight infections.

We believe that frankincense is a powerful essential oil, both for spiritual and fasting benefits. Frankincense contains pinene, which is anti-inflammatory, and it also supports the brain and nervous system. When we pray and meditate in the morning during a fast, we'll diffuse some frankincense oil to enhance the experience.

You can use it topically or diffuse it. It provides such phenomenal support for your brain and nervous system.

HOLY BASIL OIL

Holy basil has a rich history as both a therapeutic and sacred plant, with its use dating back over three thousand years. Holy basil goes by another name, "Tulsi," which means "incomparable one." The sacredness of holy basil was celebrated in the Puranas (Hindu religious texts that are part of the ancient Hindu scriptures known as the Vedas), and it is highly regarded in Ayurvedic medicine.

Numerous studies have shown eugenol, one of the chemical compounds in holy basil, to be an effective blood purifier and a heart disease deterrent.[2] Eugenol is hepatotoxic, meaning it may cause damage to the liver, which is why oils containing large percentages of eugenol should not be taken for longer than ten to fourteen days at a time.

Another compound in holy basil, caryophyllene, was found to positively impact treatments for pain, inflammation, depression, anxiety, addiction, and infections.[3] When compared with a control group, holy basil treatment proved to be a useful dietary therapy in mild to moderate non-insulin-dependent diabetes mellitus.[4]

We love to diffuse holy basil during our morning prayer and study time, particularly on fasting days, to help us focus on our goals and achieve balance.

LAVENDER OIL

When you are fasting, it's essential to keep stress hormones as low as possible and help your body relax. Lavender oil can help you do both of those things.

In quite possibly the most famous usage of all, Mary may have applied lavender with her hair to anoint Jesus. Interestingly, many researchers claim that two thousand years ago, lavender was referred to as spikenard or simply "nard" from the Greek name for lavender, *nardus*, after the Syrian city of Naarda. According to John 12:3, *"Mary took a pound of very costly oil of spikenard, anointed the feet of Jesus, and wiped His feet with her hair. And the house was filled with the fragrance of the oil."*

Today lavender oil is the most commonly used essential oil in the world. It is often considered a "must-have" oil to keep on hand at all times due to its versatile uses, including relaxing properties that promote peaceful sleep and ease feelings of tension.

The linalyl acetate found in lavender and is highly anti-inflammatory and anti-bacterial. It is also known to be calming and not prone to irritate the skin.[5]

Interestingly, a 2014 study found lavender oil not only lessened the severity of lab-induced diabetes but also improved body weight and protected the liver and kidneys from degeneration in laboratory animals.[6] So it could be a great way to enhance the detoxing effects of fasting.

We love using lavender oil topically. We also recommend taking a hot bath with Epsom salts and about twenty drops of lavender, particularly if you are on a more aggressive fasting schedule. A warm soak is profoundly relaxing and helps naturally balance hormones.

ROSEMARY OIL

Rosemary essential oil contains rosmarinic acid, which acts on the brain to improve focus, memory, and reduce inflammation. Since two of the most desirable fasting benefits are reducing inflammation and supporting brain health, rosemary oil can be a great aid during fasting.

The Ancient Egyptians, Romans, and Greeks all considered rosemary sacred, and it was widely used to cleanse the air and prevent sickness from spreading. It was used in folk medicine to improve memory, soothe digestive issues, and relieve muscle aches and pains. More recently, it has been shown to boost nerve growth factor and support the healing of neurological tissue as well as boost brain function.

Eucalyptol is a remarkable compound in rosemary that offers strong therapeutic properties. You can use it after a strenuous workout on a non-fasting day to help reduce swelling and muscle aches.[7]

A study from 2012 evaluated rosemary oil's impact on cognitive performance and mood. Twenty healthy volunteers performed tasks in a cubicle diffused with rosemary. Test results showed improved performance at higher concentrations of rosemary essential oil.[8]

We put a few drops of rosemary in a diffuser or dab two to three drops on our hands, mix it with a pinch of coconut oil, and rub it on the back of our necks to enjoy its brain-boosting and inflammation-fighting powers.

TURMERIC OIL

Turmeric is enjoying its time in the spotlight in recent years. This ancient spice, recognized for centuries as a food, medicine, and coloring agent, has experienced a surge of popularity thanks to curcumin, the therapeutic compound that supplies its brilliant yellow color.

But don't be fooled by its newfound fame; the use of turmeric dates back nearly four thousand years to the Vedic culture in India, where it was used in cooking as well as religious ceremonies. In Ayurvedic medicine, turmeric is known as strengthening and warming to the whole body.

Turmerone found in turmeric is a compound in the ketone family with many impressive benefits. For example, ar-turmerone has been found to have the ability to reduce blood sugar and induce neural stem cell growth.

There is evidence to suggest that turmerone could be a future drug candidate for treating neurological disorders, such as stroke and Alzheimer's disease. Along with turmeric's other well-studied compound, curcumin, turmerone shows promise in the area of tumor suppression.[9]

We love turmeric for its anti-inflammatory power, as well as its ability to aid with digestion and support your liver's natural detox efforts that are made more potent through fasting.

As you can see, there are many reasons to love essential oils. If you use them regularly, they can provide tremendous support during the fasting process and beyond. Experiment with different oils during fasting to see which combinations most greatly aid the experience for you.

Exogenous Ketones: The What and the Why

Researchers believe that humans developed the capacity to produce ketones (or ketone bodies) in order to prolong survival during periods of caloric deprivation.[10] Ketones are beneficial for our muscles, brains, and other tissues during times of stress—including times of "good stress," such as when you are exercising and fasting.[11]

These benefits all sound great.

So what is a ketone supplement, and should you take one while fasting?

Ketones are considered the most energy-efficient source of fuel for the body. They release high amounts of ATP (adenosine triphosphate), which is often called the "the energy currency of life." Not only can your body make ketones in response to things such as fasting or very low-carb, very high-fat dieting, but you can also acquire ketones from exogenous ketone supplements.

Exogenous ketones, such as ketone esters and BHB salts, help to amplify the many positive effects of fasting—while also mitigating potential fasting symptoms such as fatigue and brain fog. Other benefits associated with ketone supplements include:

» Helping you to shed excess weight

» Suppressing hunger and cravings

» Boosting cognitive performance

» Helping you exercise and recover more quickly

» Reducing anxiety

Ketones are formally defined as intermediate products of the breakdown of fats in the body. When you fast for an extended period (sixteen hours or more) or follow an ultra-low-carb, very high-fat diet (such as a ketogenic diet), your body starts producing organic ketone compounds, which serve as an alternative fuel source to carbohydrates.

That is why many fasters and keto dieters often take an exogenous ketone supplement to boost the effects that intermittent fasting has to offer.

Taking ketone supplements may not lead to additional weight loss if you aren't also following a low-carb or healing diet. They certainly aren't a magic bullet when it comes to weight loss, and ketones are no replacement for intermittent fasting. However, exogenous ketones can be used to help improve energy levels, power output, physical performance, and recovery from exercise.[12]

In some animal studies, researchers use ketone esters to increase rats' blood ketone levels and to test the effects on their physical performance, cardiovascular functioning, and more. In one study, when rats were given food along with a ketone ester that accounted for 30 percent of their daily calories for five days, the rats could run 32 percent farther on a treadmill compared to rats given a diet supplemented with equal amounts of corn starch or palm oil.[13]

If you find that you are having difficulty doing even light exercise while fasting, ketones may be able to help. Exogenous ketones may *increase* both exercise performance and muscle recovery.[14]

Ketones can be taken in various forms, including capsules, oils, powders, and drinks. No matter which type you use, it should be able to help raise BHB levels by supplying you with an immediate usable source of ketones. Some products will provide medium-chain triglycerides (MCTs) to help with your natural production of ketones.

Be sure to find one with no added sugar or a natural, calorie-free sweetener if you plan to take the supplement during your fasting window.

Self-Care: Mind-Body Strengthening Practices

Supplements can be a vital part of your intermittent fasting journey. However, the actions you take to better yourself and care for your mind, body, and soul are worth more than all the supplements combined.

Self-care is comprised of the actions and mindsets you employ every day that help you live your best, most vibrant life—and we believe they are a critical part of any fasting journey. First, we'll start with a brief overview of the importance of daily exercise to promote mind-body health and a positive mindset.

EXERCISE

No matter the type of exercise that fits your preferences and fasting schedule best, you're bound to experience some incredible benefits as long as you stick with it.

Dozens of protective benefits and health improvements have been associated with regular exercise in research studies. Some of these include longer lifespan, protection against heart disease and cancer, improved mental health, better sleep quality, lowered risk for obesity, reduced back pain, and protection against osteoporosis, joint pain, and osteoarthritis.[15]

Research shows that when practiced regularly, low-impact exercises such as Pilates and yoga are safe to perform while fasting and can increase flexibility, strength, length of muscles, and range of motion.[16]

Strength-building exercises are good for maintaining bone strength, protecting against falls and fractures in the elderly. When combined with a healthy diet and periodic fasting, such practices can help with weight maintenance or weight loss, especially when lifting heavier weights.

Mind-body exercises, including those that emphasize breath control while flowing through movements, are often called "moving meditations" because they can help lower stress and increase feelings of mental and even spiritual well-being. These are excellent and safe forms of exercise to utilize even during longer fasts.

For people who can handle higher impact, vigorous activities, high-intensity training offers some advantages over repeated sessions of steady-state cardio exercise—including higher calorie burn in less time, an increase in endurance, and improvements in speed and athletic performance.

Examples of high-intensity interval training exercises include sprinting alternated by periods of resting, doing a series of "burst-training" body-weight exercises, and doing CrossFit-style workouts that require lots of power output within a short period with few breaks.

However, in general, we do not recommend vigorous physical activity during an extended fasting window. Listen to your body and allow it to rest when you sense that it needs to rest.

MEDITATION

Meditation means different things to different people but usually refers to several attention-related techniques that have benefits for relieving stress and helping you stay focused and dedicated to achieving your fasting goals. Many schools of meditation have old roots in Eastern spiritual practices, but meditation is not associated with any religion and can be practiced by people of all different beliefs.

The number of studies showing benefits associated with regular meditation practice, especially the type referred to as "mindfulness meditation," has grown exponentially in recent years.

There are many different schools, definitions, and styles of meditation practiced around the world, some dating back several thousands of years. Meditation can be practiced on its own or along with some other alternative practices such as tai chi, yoga, and aromatherapy.

Although meditating doesn't always *feel* relaxing while you're doing it, research suggests that as little as ten to twenty minutes daily can be one of the best ways to control stress, anxiety, depression, lack of focus, and many other conditions. Because it helps relax the body, meditation may help address digestive disorders, acid reflux, anxiety, insomnia, high blood pressure, muscle tension, nausea due to nerves, migraines, autoimmune diseases, asthma, overeating, addictive behaviors, and others.[17]

As you may imagine, mindfulness practices can be highly beneficial when it comes to fasting as well. Meditation is associated with improved memory, attention span, happiness, sleep, hormonal balance, relationships, eating habits, weight maintenance, and blood sugar control.[18]

> Mindfulness practices can be highly beneficial when it comes to fasting as well.

A straightforward way to start practicing meditation is as follows:

1. Sit up tall with your shoulders relaxed and spine straight.
2. Lift the top of your head straight up and keep it there.
3. Inhale deeply through the nose for about four seconds and then slowly exhale out through the nose or mouth for a longer duration, about six to seven seconds.
4. Repeat as many times as desired.

Your attention and focus should stay on the feeling of the breath moving your body as much as possible. At the same time, observe any thoughts or feelings that come up without getting distracted by them. This calm observation helps relax the central nervous system and gives you something to focus on to settle your mind. Try this simple meditation practice when you are feeling the urge to snack outside your fasting window.

PRAYER

Like meditation, prayer can take many different forms. Many people begin praying during childhood and continue to do so throughout their lives, turning to spirituality and prayerful practices such as visualization or guided imagery to help them feel comforted, grateful, connected, and secure through the ups and downs in their life.

According to research regarding the power of prayer, it can also be used to help people overcome health concerns and to improve emotional and mental well-being. There's even evidence pointing to a connection between regular spiritual practice and improved health and lifespan.[19]

Hundreds of different studies have investigated the effects of prayer on various physical and mental health markers. There's some evidence that prayer can help decrease the risk for chronic diseases such as cancer, help with overcoming existing conditions and injuries, boost immune function, and improve the overall quality of life by lowering the many debilitating effects of stress.

When you focus on something other than the noise of the day, your mind will benefit. If you are fasting during the day, prayer can be the grounding force that reminds you of how fearfully and wonderfully made you are and where your strength truly comes from, which is the Lord.

Prayer takes you out of the chaos and helps increase your focus on the positive aspects of life. It can also improve your ability to carry out personal goals and fasting goals and help to form closer and more supportive relationships. It may also help to lower negative physiological processes tied to chronic worry.

> Prayer takes you out of the chaos and helps increase your focus on the positive aspects of life.

How badly do you want to be well?

How badly do you want to lose weight or be pain- and disease-free?

If you are fasting to break through to a new level of health, freedom, and happiness, we recommend that you use every single tool at your disposal. For more on the spiritual benefits of fasting, see the bonus chapter at the end of the book.

How to Set Goals and Stay Motivated

If you go into a fast without setting goals first, your chances of success are going to diminish. So, if you are committed to fasting, take the time to set goals first.

We encourage you to write down your goals for your body, mind, and spirit. We even want you to write down goals that may seem so outrageous that you are almost afraid to put them on paper.

Make sure that you write down the most significant challenges in your life and your spiritual life. This list could include emotional difficulties, family or career circumstances, weight loss, finances, personal relationships, legal situations, your children's lives, and so much more.

No one else ever has to see these goals, so don't be embarrassed. Be bold and be expectant! Write them down and watch God work each day as you give Him your time and your dedication to follow Him and stick to your fasting goals.

As a motivational tool, we also suggest that you take a before photo of your face and your body. We want you to see for yourself that your cheeks will be rosier, your eyes will be brighter, and your face and body will look far less inflamed and swollen.

Also, you should always weigh yourself the morning of your fast and then the following morning at the same time. Do this daily if it helps keep you on track. Sometimes the scale will move a lot, sometimes not at all, and sometimes in the wrong direction. Just focus on the big picture and keep weighing.

When groups fasted historically, such as the Israelites, they did it together as a people. If you don't have someone walking the fasting journey with you, rely on goals and on God to help you stay motivated to see it through!

It also wouldn't hurt to tell your family what you are doing. Share with them the goals that you are comfortable sharing and let them experience a breakthrough with you.

Who knows? Maybe you'll inspire them to start fasting as well.

Is a Cleanse Right for You?

We have mentioned throughout the book that some "fasts" could also include vegetable juices and bone broth.

Wait—but don't those have calories?

Yes, but there are still advantages to liquid cleanses that we will quickly address.

VEGETABLE JUICE CLEANSE

Juice cleanses have spent a long time now in the limelight. From boutique juice shops to social media stars broadcasting their juice cleanse before and after photos all over Instagram, no doubt juicing is widespread and only seems to be growing in popularity.

Is juicing as good for you as its fans seem to think? And how does it compare to fasting in terms of benefits?

First, let's define what we mean by juice cleanse. A juice cleanse involves drinking juices made from fruits and vegetables for a specific window of time. In some cases, this can be as simple as sipping on a glass of celery juice each morning. It could also involve nixing all other foods and consuming only juice during your "cleansing" time.

There are many different types of juice cleanses out there. One of the most popular methods involves purchasing store-bought juices and following a premade plan from companies such as Suja Juice.

While store-bought juices are certainly healthier than 100 percent fruit juices and juices from concentrate, if you want to do a juice cleanse for healing purposes, we recommend making your own with a juicer. Making homemade juice offers you more flexibility and allows you to select ingredients targeted to your specific needs.

The duration of a cleanse can also range a great deal, from just a few days to several weeks at a time. There are a few key benefits to juice cleansing:

1. *Juice cleansing provides a burst of micronutrients.* How many of us eat the seven servings of vegetables daily that

are recommended to promote better health and prevent chronic disease? Very few people do. Juicing provides you with tons of nutrients in an easy-to-consume form.

2. *Juice cleansing enhances nutrient absorption.* Drinking juice is like taking a shot of instant nutrition goodness. Because all the insoluble fiber has been removed through the juicing process, digestion becomes a lot easier on the body.

3. *Juice cleansing complements other wellness protocols.* Gerson cancer therapy protocols, for example, call for thirteen, eight-ounce glasses of juice every day.

One potential downside to juicing is you may not lose as much weight as you think you might. If you're planning on going on a juice cleanse to lose weight, take note that you might find yourself feeling hungry a lot more often. Solid foods help you reach satiety and feel fuller than drinking your meals. So if you're regularly drinking juices, you might find yourself eating more food—and drinking more calories—more often to feel satisfied. This tendency is particularly true if you include lots of fruit juices in your cleanse (which we do not recommend).

Additionally, juicing can get expensive. Even if you're making homemade juice, you often need double or triple the amount of ingredients to make one juice compared to if you ate the food whole. If you buy fresh, organic produce, those numbers start to add up quickly, particularly if the entire family is enjoying juices as well.

If you decide to do a juice cleanse, we don't recommend including any fruit juices aside from lemons and limes. A little bit of freshly pressed apple juice is OK, but the primary juices should be from vegetables.

Carrot juice is nutritious and tasty, but carrots do contain more sugar than other veggies, so they shouldn't be your base juice. Beets are also super-nutritious but higher in sugar, so limit your carrot and beet juices to 25 percent of total juice. We prefer juices made with celery, cucumber, greens, cilantro, parsley, lemons, limes, ginger root, and turmeric root.

When we do a juice cleanse, we like to drink a large glass of juice at regular breakfast, lunch, and dinner times, but you can experiment with the timing to see what works best for you. Some people sip on their juice all day long. Drinking juice throughout the day is only advisable if your juices are extremely low in sugar.

A juice fast or cleanse is particularly beneficial when dealing with acute illness as well as a disease such as cancer. Juice cleanses are also fantastic for your skin.

Along with the juices, you may also wish to drink herbal teas made with ashwagandha, astragalus, turmeric, ginger, and cinnamon. These contain different types of powerful cancer-fighting, fat-burning, and hormone-balancing nutrients.

We've seen juice cleanses transform lives when they are done correctly. And for many, they are far more doable than a water-only fast.

A lot of people are nutritionally bankrupt, with low levels of vitamins and minerals. Juice cleanses flood your body, your organs, and your cells with nutrients. If you are feeling drained and depleted, a boost of nutrients in the form of a juice cleanse may be just what you need.

BONE BROTH CLEANSE

The second type of cleanse we want to discuss is the bone broth cleanse or diet.

The bone broth diet is a popular eating plan that combines the principles of intermittent fasting and the healing diet while also allowing you to take advantage of the benefits of bone broth. The basics of the plan are as follows.

First, you select a length of time, such as twenty-one days, to do the cleanse. During that period, you drink one to three servings of bone broth per day, alongside a diet rich in whole, unprocessed foods for five days per week. It's also advisable to avoid grains, gluten, soy, dairy, and sugar during this time.

Then, for the remaining two days a week, you consume only bone broth for all of your snacks and meals throughout the day.

So we suppose you could call it with Paleo/healing diet–based 5:2 plan with bone broth added to the fasting days.

Many people use the bone broth diet for weight loss. The plan swaps out processed foods for nutritious whole foods while also bumping up your intake of protein, which has been shown to reduce appetite and caloric intake to support weight loss.[20] It also involves intermittent fasting, which means you get the benefits of the bone broth, the healing foods, and fasting, all in one plan.

Proponents of the plan say it may also help:

» **Reduce inflammation**. The plan works by pairing bone broth—an ingredient that contains anti-inflammatory compounds like collagen—with intermittent fasting, a practice you now know has also been linked to decrease markers of inflammation.[21]

» **Promote gut health**. The bone broth diet is also said to support gut health and protect against leaky gut syndrome.

» **Improve joint function**. If you suffer from chronic joint pain, swelling, or stiffness, adding bone broth to your routine may be beneficial. This is because it's a great source of collagen, which helps restore cartilage and keep the joints healthy.

» **Keep skin healthy**. Bone broth may help slow the signs of aging to keep skin healthy and hydrated. Studies show that collagen could improve skin elasticity and moisture in older women.[22]

For most healthy adults, the bone broth diet is safe and associated with minimal adverse side effects. To determine if the diet is right for you, try following a seven-day bone broth diet plan to see how you feel.

However, the bone broth diet may not be right for everyone. Women who are pregnant and nursing, for example, should not follow the bone broth diet and should instead focus on consuming a well-rounded, nutrient-rich diet. Those with underlying health conditions such as diabetes or kidney disease should consult with their doctors before considering the bone broth diet.

You Can Do All Things

We would never pretend for a moment that fasting and cleansing are easy for everyone. We're not big coffee drinkers, so it's easy for us to say, "Don't drink coffee." But if you have been dealing with food addiction for any amount of time, you know that self-control and discipline when it comes to eating is undoubtedly no easy thing.

It's also easy for people who regularly fast and exercise to tell someone else, "C'mon, it's good for you. Just do it."

The story is never that black and white, and nothing is ever that clear cut. However, there is one thing that we know for sure is real for everyone reading this book. Christ can give you the strength to do anything you truly wish to do in your life.

> "I can do **all** things through Christ who strengthens me" (**Philippians 4:13**).

If you are struggling with where to start or what step to take first, let us make it simple for you: First, pray about it.

Then, if you are ready to give fasting a try, don't eat anything after dinner tonight. Then, tomorrow morning, wait just one hour longer than you usually do to eat breakfast.

That's all we ask—just two things. Skip evening snacking and wait one more hour to have breakfast. If you can do that, you can eventually work toward any time-restricted eating goal you have.

Losing weight, reversing premature aging, and healing from within are not easy tasks. If these goals were effortless to accomplish, we wouldn't have the immense pain and suffering in this country that we currently face from lifestyle-related diseases.

> You can reach your ideal
> weight. You can feel
> vibrant and youthful again.
> You can heal your gut,
> reduce inflammation,
> destroy tumors, unlock
> limitless energy, and break
> addictions.

You can reach your ideal weight. You can feel vibrant and youthful again. You can heal your gut, reduce inflammation, destroy tumors, unlock limitless energy, and break addictions. All of this and more can be manifested in your life, if you will take the time and have the discipline to fast and cleanse.

Blessings to you on your fasting journey!

BONUS

THE SPIRITUAL BENEFITS OF FASTING

Fasting for Spiritual Breakthrough

We saved the best for last.

Fasting can be one of the best things you will ever do for your body, but it can also be a life-changing experience for you and your walk with God as well. He can show you ways to break through strongholds in your life that you would have never believed could be defeated.

Whenever you start a fast, keep this cautioning found in Ephesians 6:12 in mind: *"For our struggle is not against flesh and blood, but against the rulers, against the authorities, against the powers of this dark world and against the spiritual forces of evil in the heavenly realms"* (NIV).

When you undergo a fast, the enemy knows you are about to have an incredible discovery in your life, and he wants to stop it. Here are some of the challenges that you may face during a fast that you undertake for spiritual purposes, such as a ten-day Daniel Fast:

ON THE SPIRITUAL SIDE

Circumstances in your life may seem to be impossible to overcome. This means the fast is working. The temptation to break the fast may seem to increase, and you may come up with several "good" reasons to stop it. This means the fast is working.

ON THE EMOTIONAL SIDE

Because your body will begin throwing off deadly emotions, an initial increase in nervousness, anxiety, and worry may result. This means the fast is working.

ON THE PHYSICAL SIDE

Since your body will begin to detoxify, you may experience a coated tongue, headaches, bad breath, body odor, digestion and elimination changes, mild fatigue, and possibly even the sniffles. This means the fast is working.

> Fasting can be one of the best things you will ever do for your body, but it can also be a life-changing experience for you and your walk with God as well.

Fasting allows you to receive breakthrough in areas of your life that simply cannot be accomplished any other way.

If you look up *fasting* in the dictionary, you'll see the definition is "to go without food," but we believe, as our ancestors did and as Jesus Himself did, that fasting can be so much more than that.

If you need a spiritual awakening or to hear from God, the answer is fasting. It allows you to receive breakthrough in areas of your life that simply cannot be accomplished any other way. That must be why the great men and women of God and the Son of God chose not only to pray but also to fast.

Remember that intensity you felt when you first got saved? Is it still there? If it's not, fasting can rekindle your fire and your passion for growing closer to Christ once again.

Now you can't just fast to *force* God to do something, and you can't just fast to get a physical benefit or believe you are somehow "entitled" to a breakthrough. You have to fast and devote your time and your body to God, expecting nothing in return but yet remaining open to possibility and fully expecting Him to bring about *His* will for your life.

> Fasting can rekindle your fire and your passion for growing closer to Christ once again.

The Fab Four and a Bold Request

Let's talk a little bit more about the young man Daniel, and his three friends Hananiah, Azariah, and Mishael. These four Jews were taken into captivity at the great siege of Jerusalem, where King Nebuchadnezzar and his army brought people from Israel to be enslaved in Babylon.

There's every indication that this quartet was treated well because they were seen as assets by the king's court. They were the best of the best, the crème de la crème who, were they alive today, would have gotten perfect 2400 scores on their SATs or aced their law school entrance exam.

Think National Merit Scholars.

Biblical academics believe the fab four were around fourteen years old when they were placed under the guidance of Ashpenaz, who was in charge of the palace personnel, to teach them the Chaldean language and literature. Like hotshot recruits entering college, they were assigned the best foods from the king's own kitchen during their training period. Nothing would be spared for these elite scholars who looked—as well as acted—the part.

Daniel and his three friends may have grown up in spiritually depraved Judah, but somebody in their lives (a parent, an uncle, a rabbi, or a prophet) must have modeled how they should serve God. That's the best explanation we have for why they refused to eat the rich foods set before them at the king's table.

You see, these "foods" were considered detestable to the God of Heaven whom they faithfully served. Perhaps they were presented with meats that had been sacrificed to idols, or meats that were unclean because the animals had been strangled or contaminated with blood or fat—or all of the above.

More likely, though, they were offered meats that God forbade His people to eat in Leviticus 11 and Deuteronomy 14. We're talking about pork, rabbits, camels, badgers, snakes, and flesh-eating birds such as vultures.

Shellfish was also unclean according to the ancient law, but it's doubtful that lobster or scampi were on King Nebuchadnezzar's menu because Babylon was too far away from a saltwater ocean. But they could have been served catfish, eel, or other smooth-skinned species that were also off-limits according to God's commands.

Daniel also passed on the king's wine. While there was no scriptural injunction against drinking wine, perhaps Daniel knew the pitfalls that awaited those consuming excess alcohol and wanted to present his body to God as a living sacrifice.

The desire to obey God and treat his body like a temple prompted him to make the request: "Please give us only water to drink and pulse to eat and test us in this. See if, after ten days, we do not have greater physical strength, health, and appearance." (See Dan. 1:12–13.)

For a young man to utter those words—that's more than bold.

By now, you know how the story ends. After just ten days, they looked better and performed better than all the other boys. They were found to have a more exceptional physical appearance, greater wisdom, and superior health.

God bestowed on them and multiplied upon them during those ten days. They had so much faith in their God that when Daniel's three friends, later renamed Shadrach, Meshach, and Abed-Nego, were asked to bow to an idol or be thrown in the firing furnace, they said, "Our God will deliver us, but even if He doesn't, we will never bow." (See Dan. 3:17–18.)

Oh, that we would all have that kind of faith!

Spiritual Revolutions Await

Most Christians we meet and other fasting enthusiasts are interested in the benefits of the Daniel Fast, which is why we want to emphasize that the Daniel Fast can be so much more than just a *natural* way to look and feel better.

We consider the Daniel Fast to be a divine or *supernatural* health plan that combines the Bible's ancient wisdom and the best of modern science. In the same way that the king and his men were shocked at Daniel's and his friends' transformation, we've been in awe of the change we've seen in people who do the Daniel Fast for just ten days.

> The Daniel Fast is a divine or ***supernatural*** health plan that combines the Bible's ancient wisdom and the best of modern science.

We've seen twenty pounds gone in days. We've seen addictions broken. We've seen relationships healed. In both of our lives, we've personally experienced God's power through both natural medicine and supernatural healing.

We believe that there are immense physical, emotional, and spiritual benefits to fasting. The benefits of fasting for a spiritual breakthrough are many, but we feel the top four spiritual reasons to fast are:

1. FASTING CAN BRING YOU CLOSER TO GOD.

Fasting can undeniably bring you closer to God. Isaiah 58:9 says that you will call on the Lord and He will say, *"Here I am."* When you give Him the control of your most primitive desire (hunger) and focus on God, the distance between you is significantly reduced. You will have a relationship with God that you never thought possible because you are giving up what is most important to the human body—and God knows it.

2. FASTING CAN MAKE YOU MORE SENSITIVE TO GOD'S VOICE.

When you begin to orient your life around God's plan, you begin to hear Him. You may be thinking, "I've never heard God. I read about God. I know who God is, but hearing Him?" We believe that God will speak to you during your fast. You will hear His still and small voice and know it's God. He will move you to do things that you couldn't think of on your own. He will give you abilities that you never had before.

3. FASTING HELPS BREAK ADDICTIONS.

The lust of the flesh is intense, and this world is filled with temptation. There are gambling and pornography. There are drugs and alcohol. There is also food addiction. When you give up the physical desire to eat, strongholds will begin to be broken, and yokes will be broken as well.

4. FASTING SHOWS US OUR WEAKNESS AND ALLOWS US TO RELY ON GOD'S STRENGTH.

We are all sinners. It's always good to be reminded of this and to remember from whom our strength comes. Fasting will also help you see that creator God made no mistakes when He made you. You are perfect and perfectly His.

Fasting can help relieve anxiety, nervousness, and even fear. Fasting can also help ease depression and clear your mind of negative thoughts. Fasting brings peace. When you give up your most significant appetite to God, He will allow you to break free. He will enable you to take your thoughts captive and renew your mind.

Fasting can help relieve anxiety, nervousness, and even fear. Fasting can also help ease depression and clear your mind of negative thoughts. Fasting brings peace.

Philippians 4:6-7 says, *"Do not be anxious about anything, but in every situation, by prayer and petition, with thanksgiving, present your requests to God. And the peace of God, which transcends all understanding, will guard your hearts and your minds in Christ Jesus"* (NIV).

Let us tell you that fasting in this manner is worth every hunger pang and every doubt, so ask God to give you the strength and the desire to fast for a breakthrough.

There Is Power in the Name

When you fast and pray—two words that go hand in hand in Scripture—you pursue God in your life and open yourself up to experiencing a renewed dependence on God, but it isn't easy. It is a spiritual discipline that requires denying your physical and mental self, because your stomach and your brain will most likely work overtime to remind you when and what they want to eat.

Here are some questions to ask yourself as you consider whether now might be the right time to engage in the Daniel Fast:

» Do I need God's hand to touch my life?

» Do I need a healing miracle?

» Am I fearful of the world or current events?

- » Do I desire a deeper relationship with God?
- » Do I feel shackled by bondages that I cannot escape?
- » Am I in a toxic relationship, and I don't know what to do?
- » Do I have a friend or loved one who needs salvation?
- » Am I ready to find what plans God has next for my life?
- » Do I feel distant from God, and I'm not sure why?

Before you begin your fast, you can make a list of prayer requests you are asking God to answer. Then, every time you experience hunger pangs or food or drink cravings, ask God to work in your Daniel Fast prayer request areas.

The Daniel Fast requires you to eat a vegan diet for ten days. Now we are both personally omnivores. Jesus consumed animal foods, and we have reason to believe that all the disciples did. But for ten days, Daniel and his friends consumed pulse and water. If you also eat in this manner for ten days, God will do supernatural things in your body, mind, and spirit.

God gave us three governing principles to follow on this fast:

1. Eat only what God created for food.
2. Eat food in a form that is healthy for the body and don't try to alter God's design.
3. Don't make any food or drink your idol. We idolize caffeinated beverages. We idolize alcoholic drinks. People worship at the table where we eat—and that is not the kind of worship God wants.

Follow these guidelines and submit to God, and we will launch you into a lifestyle of healthy eating and living, with revelations that you've never heard before.

If you find yourself struggling to keep your eyes fixed on Jesus, we encourage you to go to the Word and read. Hebrews 12:1–2 reminds us, *"Let us throw off everything that hinders and the sin that so easily entangles. And let us run with perseverance the race marked out for us, fixing our eyes on Jesus, the pioneer and perfecter of faith"* (NIV).

If you feel negativity or doubt creep in, speak words of life over yourself and your fast. Read Romans 8:28: *"And we know that God causes everything to work together for the good of those who love God and are called according to his purpose for them"* (NLT).

Here are some other positive affirmations that you can use to speak life into your body, your finances, your family, your career, and your spirit.

- » In the name of Jesus, I refuse every negative word and opinion working against me.
- » In the name of Jesus, I claim healing over my body.
- » In the name of Jesus, every power against me is dismantled by God's grace in my life.
- » In the name of Jesus, my body is blessed because I choose to walk in obedience.
- » In the name of Jesus, every financial mismanagement that is hindering my prosperity is released.

We recommend that while you are following the Daniel Fast you spend quiet time with God each day, reading Scripture and journaling your thoughts and your victories, both big and small. Let this be a time of personal awakening. Each day write down the areas of your life where you can feel God working.

We worship the living God. Remember that He is with you and has not forgotten you. Fasting could be the catalyst you need to draw closer to Him.

When in doubt, just say His name! There is power in the name of Jesus.

> We worship the living God. Remember that He is with you and has not forgotten you. Fasting could be the catalyst you need to draw closer to Him.

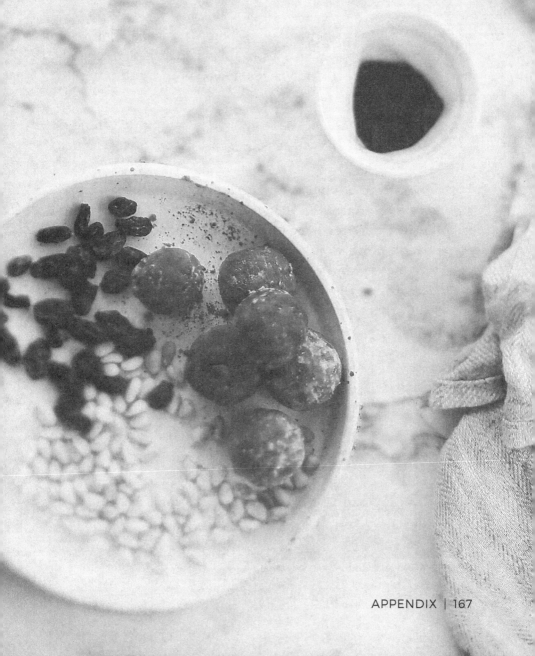

APPENDIX

Sample 18:6 Time-Restricted Eating Plan

As we have said many times before, there is no single right way to fast! It's important to design a fasting plan and an eating schedule that fits you and your unique needs, as well as any health concerns you may have.

To get you started, we have created a sample 18:6 time-restricted eating plan that you can customize according to your daily schedule.

For those who are brand new to fasting, we recommend you start with a 12:12 plan and progress from there, at the pace that feels right for you. If you need to extend your eating window, adjust these eating times to fit with your goals, tolerance, and health concerns. This is only a suggestion, and if you have any preexisting conditions, please talk to a medical health professional (we recommend a functional medicine practitioner) to ensure that this plan is suitable for you.

- » 6:00 a.m. Wake up and super-hydrate with a large glass of water.
- » 6:00–7:00 a.m. Work out, pray, meditate (drink plenty of water).
- » 7:00–8:00 a.m. Shower, get ready for the day, commute to work.
- » 8:00–12:00 p.m. Drink water, unsweetened herbal teas, coffee.

» 12:00–1:00 p.m. Eat lunch! Eat until full and don't count calories. Follow the healing diet guidelines and use the recipes in this book.

» 1:00–3:00 p.m. Drink water and unsweetened drinks.

» 3:00–3:15 p.m. If feeling hungry, have some kombucha or bone broth. If you need to eat some food because you are feeling sluggish or dizzy, opt for fresh fruit or a healthy fat (nuts, nut butter, avocado).

» 5:00–6:00 Eat dinner! Eat until full and don't count calories. Feel free to enjoy a sweet treat such as a bowl of strawberries or try one of our dessert recipes in this book.

Follow this plan two or three more times a week for a month and experience dramatic breakthroughs in your life and your health!

A Quick Guide to Macronutrient Deficiency

One of the issues often faced with IMF is people get into "food ruts" and consume the same few foods over and over again. While this may be convenient, it can also lead to macronutrient deficiencies.

When someone does not get enough of a particular macronutrient or gets too much of only one kind, dysfunction and disease is more likely to occur. Even if a serious condition doesn't occur due to imbalances in macronutrient intake, noticeable and lingering symptoms are still possible. The following table provides you with risks associated with eating too little of each of the big three macronutrients.

INSUFFICIENT PROTEIN

» A sluggish metabolism and trouble losing weight

» Low energy levels, weakness, and fatigue

» Poor concentration and trouble learning

» Moodiness, anxiety, and mood swings

» Muscle, bone, and joint pain

» Blood sugar changes that can lead to diabetes

» Lowered immunity

INSUFFICIENT FAT

» Poor brain function

» Compromised heart health

» Hormone imbalances

» Weight gain

» Higher risk of insulin resistance and diabetes

» Higher risk for depression and anxiety

» Gut-related problems

INSUFFICIENT CARBS (FRUITS AND VEGGIES)

» Low energy levels, weakness, and fatigue

» Carb and sugar cravings

» Constipation or bloating due to water retention

» Diminished athletic performance

» Trouble sleeping

» Moodiness or irritability

» Loss of libido

» Skin dryness and hair thinning

A Quick Guide to Micronutrient Whole Food Sources

No one can deny that vitamins and minerals (micronutrients) are essential. Sadly, most diets are extremely deficient in micronutrients. While supplementation can be helpful, there is nothing quite like taking in essential nutrients in whole food form. The "right" amount of macronutrients in one's diet depends on specific goals, medical history, level of activity, and many other factors. Use this guide to discover how to naturally take in the micronutrients your body needs.

Type of Food	Examples	Micronutrient Benefits
Green Leafy Vegetables	Kale, collard greens, spinach, bok choy, cabbage, lettuces, and Swiss chard	» Excellent sources of vitamin C, vitamin A, vitamin K, folic acid, and magnesium
Starchy and Non-Starchy Vegetables	Red peppers, broccoli, squash, cauliflower, green peppers, artichokes, carrots, asparagus, tomatoes, and mushrooms	» Great for providing fiber, magnesium, potassium, vitamin A and vitamin C

Fruits	Strawberries, blueberries, raspberries, melon, pineapple, bananas, apples, pears, and kiwi	» High in antioxidants such as vitamin A and C, fiber, and potassium » Berries are associated with brain health and cancer prevention » Many berries are high in quercetin, a protective phytonutrient that fights inflammation
Nuts and Seeds	Chia seeds, flax, hemp, pecans, almonds, walnuts, macadamia nuts, and sunflower seeds	» Provide antioxidants such as vitamin E and micronutrients such as selenium, zinc, magnesium, boron, and choline » Good sources of omega-3 fatty acids, fiber, and some protein
High-Quality Animal Products	Wild seafood, cage-free eggs, grass-fed beef, and pasture-raised poultry	» Excellent sources iron, B vitamins, vitamin A, and zinc » Organ meats are especially dense in B vitamins, iron, and vitamin A » Cage-free eggs offer multiple nutrients, including choline, vitamin A, and vitamin E » Dairy products such as milk, cheese and yogurt provide B vitamins, iron, calcium, and potassium

Type of Food	Examples	Micronutrient Benefits
Beans and Legumes	Peas, green beans, kidney beans, black beans, lentils, snap peas, navy beans, bean sprouts	» High in calcium, manganese, folate, phosphorus and iron » Excellent sources of fiber, and therefore great for promoting digestion and controlling cholesterol
100 Percent Whole Grains	100 percent whole wheat and ancient grains such as quinoa, amaranth, oats, and buckwheat	» Provide B vitamins and minerals such as iron, manganese, and phosphorus » Compared to processed grains, they are higher in essential nutrients, fiber, and protein

Overall, if you eat a variety of fresh foods, you will be well on your way to acquiring enough micronutrients. Organic, fresh foods are more likely to contain higher amounts of micronutrients compared to processed foods, foods grown in depleted soil, or those that have been sitting on store shelves for an extended period of time.

A Quick Guide to the Healing Diet

The Healing Foods Diet is rich in nutritious whole foods from the earth. Grass-fed meat, wild-caught fish, and organic poultry and eggs are also permitted as part of the plan, along with an assortment of healthy condiments, herbs, and spices. Whether or not you are fasting, we recommend using the following lists to guide your diet and eating philosophies.

What to eat (not an exhaustive list but good suggestions):

» **Fruits:** strawberries, oranges, lemons, blackberries, limes, raspberries, pears, apples, blueberries, watermelon, kiwi, grapefruit

» **Vegetables:** broccoli, kale, spinach, cabbage, bell peppers, brussels sprouts, tomatoes, asparagus, cucumber, onions, ginger, zucchini, greens, cauliflower

» **Nuts:** almonds, cashews, pecans, pistachios, macadamia nuts, walnuts, Brazil nuts

» **Seeds:** hemp seeds, pumpkin seeds, sunflower seeds, chia seeds, flaxseeds

» **Legumes:** black beans, kidney beans, pinto beans, lima beans, chickpeas, lentils

» **Whole grains:** quinoa, barley, buckwheat, millet, brown rice

» **Healthy fats:** olive oil, coconut oil, MCT oil, grass-fed butter, ghee, avocado oil

- » **Dairy products:** goat milk, kefir, goat cheese, probiotic yogurt, raw milk
- » **Meat:** grass-fed beef, lamb, venison, wild game
- » **Fish:** wild-caught salmon, tuna, mackerel, anchovies, sardines
- » **Poultry:** organic chicken, turkey, goose, duck
- » **Eggs:** cage-free, free-range, organic (and ideally pasture-raised) eggs
- » **Condiments:** hummus, guacamole, apple cider vinegar, mustard, salsa, balsamic vinegar, liquid aminos
- » **Herbs and spices:** ginger, garlic, basil, oregano, rosemary, turmeric, cinnamon, paprika, cumin, black pepper
- » **Natural sweeteners:** stevia, raw honey, maple syrup, dates, monk fruit
- » **Beverages:** water, tea, organic coffee, kombucha, bone broth

Just as important as filling up on the right foods is limiting your consumption of unhealthy, pro-inflammatory ingredients. Not only are these foods typically high in calories, sodium, and added sugars, they can also contribute to the development of chronic disease.

What to remove:

- » **Refined grains:** white rice, pasta, white bread, breakfast cereals
- » **Added sugars:** soda, juice, candies, cookies, granola bars, baked goods, ice cream
- » **Unhealthy fats:** refined vegetable oils, shortening, hydrogenated fats, fried foods
- » **Conventional meat and poultry**

» **Farmed fish**

» **Processed foods:** potato chips, crackers, frozen meals, microwave popcorn, processed meat, instant noodles

Healing Diet and Daniel Fast Recipes

This recipe collection was designed to provide you with delicious, filling options for your daily eating window or even when you are not fasting!

The goal is to fill you up with nutrient-dense meals that are made with whole, nutrient-dense foods.

If a recipe is vegan, Paleo, or gluten-free, it is listed as such. If you have dairy sensitivities to raw cheeses or other food sensitivities or allergies, you can substitute as needed.

Pro Tip: Coconuts and cashews in their many forms provide numerous substitution options for those who are vegan or nondairy.

RECIPE CATEGORIES

- » Breakfast
- » Main Dishes
- » Side Dishes
- » Desserts
- » Beverages and Smoothies
- » Soups
- » Daniel Fast Friendly Meals

Tropical Acai Bowl with Mango and Hemp Seeds

Vegan, Paleo, Gluten-Free

Serves 3–4

Ingredients

1 fresh mango or papaya, cubed

3 frozen bananas, sliced

½ cup frozen berries (of choice)

1 cup acai concentrate

Toppings

Hemp seeds

Chia seeds

Desiccated coconut

Sliced kiwi

Fresh blueberries

Granola or pumpkin seeds

Directions

1. Add everything to a blender, blending on medium-high until thick and creamy.

2. Evenly distribute mixture into 2–3 bowls and top with toppings.

Crustless Spinach Quiche

Gluten-Free

Serves 4

Ingredients

1 tablespoon coconut oil + extra for greasing

1 onion, chopped

1 package frozen chopped spinach, thawed and drained

8 eggs, beaten

1½ cups shredded raw cheese

¼ teaspoon sea salt

⅛ teaspoon black pepper

Directions

1. Preheat oven to 350 degrees F and grease a 9-inch pie pan with coconut oil.
2. Heat coconut oil and onions over medium heat in saucepan until onions are soft. Stir in spinach and cook until excess moisture has evaporated.
3. In a bowl, combine eggs, cheese, salt and pepper. Stir.
4. Add spinach mixture and mix together.
5. Scoop into pan and bake for 30 minutes.

Apple Cinnamon Baked Oatmeal

Gluten-Free

Serves 6

Ingredients

4 cups full-fat, canned coconut milk

½ cup coconut sugar

2 tablespoons butter

½ teaspoon sea salt

¼ teaspoon nutmeg

⅛ teaspoon cardamom

¾ teaspoon cinnamon

2 cups steel cut oats

2 cups chopped apples

½ cup raisins

1 cup chopped nuts

Directions

1. Preheat oven to 350 F.
2. Bring coconut milk, coconut sugar, butter, salt, nutmeg, cardamom, and cinnamon to boil in pot over high heat.
3. Add remaining ingredients to pot and mix.
4. Transfer contents to greased Dutch oven and bake for 30–35 minutes.

Chocolate Banana Muffins

Gluten-Free

Serves 12

Ingredients

½ cup butter, softened

1 cup coconut sugar

2 eggs

1 cup ripe bananas, mashed

2/3 cup sprouted almond butter

1 tablespoon coconut milk

1 teaspoon vanilla extract

2 cups gluten-free flour

1 teaspoon baking soda

½ teaspoon sea salt

¾ cup dark chocolate chips

Directions

1. Preheat the oven to 375 degrees F.
2. In a bowl, mix the butter and sugar until well combined.
3. Add in the eggs, one at a time.
4. Beat in bananas, almond butter, coconut milk, and vanilla.
5. In a separate bowl, combine the flour, baking soda and salt.
6. Combine both bowls and fold in the chips.
7. Fill tins with cupcake liners and add the dough until ¾ full and bake for 18–25 minutes.

Slow Cooker Breakfast Casserole

Gluten-Free

Serves 4

Ingredients

12 eggs

½ cup goat kefir

½ teaspoon red pepper flakes

1 teaspoon sea salt

½ teaspoon black pepper

1 cup raw goat cheese, shredded

1 cup raw sheep cheese, shredded

½ cup green onions, chopped

2 sweet potatoes, peeled and grated into hash browns

1 pound chicken sausage, chopped

½ cup bell pepper, chopped

Directions

1. In a bowl, beat eggs, kefir, red pepper flakes, salt, and pepper. Stir in half the goat cheese, half the sheep cheese, and half the green onions.

2. In a medium bowl, mix together the potatoes, sausage, peppers, remaining cheese and onions. Add to slow cooker.

3. Pour egg mixture over layers and cook on low for 6–8 hours.

French Toast with Sourdough

Serves 2–4

Ingredients

½ loaf crusty sourdough bread

5 eggs

1 cup coconut milk

1 tablespoon vanilla extract

1 tablespoon cinnamon

6 tablespoons ghee

Directions

1. Slice the bread into 8 slices.
2. In a medium bowl, whisk together the eggs, milk, vanilla, and cinnamon. Drench the bread in the mixture, allowing it to soak for 2 minutes per piece.
3. Heat a skillet over medium-high heat. Add 1 tablespoon of ghee to the skillet.
4. Working in batches of 1–2 slices each, fry the drenched bread until crispy, 3–4 minutes per side. Add more ghee to the skillet in between batches.
5. Serve hot with butter and maple syrup or fruit.

Veggie Omelet

Paleo, Gluten-Free

Serves 1–2

Ingredients

3 eggs, whisked

1 garlic clove, chopped

½ cup chopped red pepper

½ cup chopped green pepper

½ cup chopped mushrooms

¼ cup chopped red onion

2 tablespoons grass-fed butter

2 ounces raw goat or sheep cheese

Oregano, chives, black pepper, and sea salt to taste

Directions

1. Sauté garlic, peppers, mushrooms, onion, and butter in a saucepan over medium-low heat.
2. After 5 minutes, add eggs.
3. Shred the cheese on top and fold into an omelet.
4. Serve with oregano, chives, black pepper, and sea salt.

Breakfast Quesadilla

Gluten-Free (unless using Ezekiel tortillas)

Serves 2

Ingredients

4 brown rice, grain-free or Ezekiel tortillas

¼ cup sprouted almond butter

1 peach, peeled and diced

1 pear, peeled and diced

1 tablespoon raw honey

Cinnamon to taste

1 tablespoon coconut oil

Directions

1. On the center of a tortilla, spread almond butter and top with the diced peaches and pears.

2. Drizzle the fruit with honey and sprinkle cinnamon on top.

3. Place a second tortilla on top.

4. In a large skillet over medium heat, melt coconut oil or butter.

5. Place quesadilla in the skillet, flipping once, until both sides are golden brown and crispy. Repeat with remaining tortillas.

6. Drizzle with honey and serve.

Almond Berry Cereal

Vegan, Paleo, Gluten-Free

Serves 1

Ingredients

3 tablespoons almonds

4 tablespoons coconut milk

4 tablespoons flax meal

½ cup blueberries

1 teaspoon cinnamon

Directions

1. Put almonds, coconut milk, flax meal, blueberries in a bowl.
2. Sprinkle with cinnamon.

Flourless Pancakes

Paleo, Gluten-Free

Serves 1

Ingredients

2 ripe bananas, mashed

3 eggs

1 teaspoon cinnamon

1 teaspoon vanilla extract

Sea salt to taste

Ghee

Directions

1. Thoroughly combine all ingredients in a bowl.
2. Place several large spoonfuls of batter spread out in the skillet pan with melted ghee over medium heat.
3. Cook until small bubbles form and then flip.

Buffalo Chicken Tenders

Paleo, Gluten-Free

Serves 2

Ingredients

- 1 pound chicken tender strips
- ½ cup cassava flour
- ½ teaspoon paprika
- ¼ teaspoon cayenne pepper
- ¼ teaspoon sea salt
- ¼ teaspoon black pepper
- ¼ teaspoon garlic powder
- ½ cup hot sauce, plus more to taste
- 2 tablespoons coconut oil
- ¼ cup ghee

Directions

1. Cut all chicken strips in half.
2. In a medium bowl, combine cassava flour, paprika, cayenne pepper, sea salt, pepper, and garlic powder.
3. In a separate bowl, pour in hot sauce.
4. Melt coconut oil in pan over medium heat.
5. Coat both sides of chicken with flour mixture.
6. Dip floured chicken in hot sauce.
7. Place all in pan and cook for 6–7 minutes.
8. Add butter to pan and flip the chicken.
9. Cook second side for 6–7 minutes until cooked through.
10. Remove from heat and add additional hot sauce as needed.
11. Serve hot.

Easy Margherita Pizza
(for Those Busy Weeknights)

Gluten-Free

Serves 8–10

Ingredients

1 flatbread pizza crust (gluten-free store bought or make your own)

1/3 – ½ cup pizza sauce

1 8-ounce container buffalo mozzarella

6–8 grape tomatoes, halved lengthwise

2 cloves garlic, minced

Fresh basil, chiffonade, for topping

Red pepper flakes, for topping (optional)

Directions

1. Preheat oven to 400°F.
2. Place all toppings on the baked flatbread pizza crust and bake for 15 minutes.
3. Top with crushed red pepper.

Slow Cooker Beef Stew

Paleo, Gluten-Free
Serves 5–6

Ingredients

2 pounds grass-fed beef stew meat
4 carrots, coarsely chopped
2 parsnips, coarsely chopped
2 cups beef broth
2 tablespoons Worcestershire sauce
2 tablespoons balsamic vinegar
6 ounces tomato paste
2 cups fire-roasted tomatoes
1 cup mushrooms, sliced
1 onion, sliced
1 teaspoon garlic powder
1 teaspoon onion powder
1 teaspoon smoked paprika
2 tablespoons fresh dill, chopped
3 sprigs thyme
3 bay leaves
2 tablespoons avocado oil
4 tablespoons arrowroot starch
1 teaspoon sea salt
1 teaspoon black pepper
Parsley, for garnishing

Directions

1. Place all ingredients into a slow cooker except for the parsley.

2. Cook on low for 6–8 hours.

3. Top with chopped parsley and serve.

Moo Shu Chicken Lettuce Wraps

Paleo, Gluten-Free

Serves 6–8

Ingredients

1 tablespoon sesame oil

2 tablespoons balsamic vinegar

2 tablespoons coconut aminos

1 teaspoon ginger, grated

2 cloves garlic, minced

½ teaspoon sea salt

½ teaspoon black pepper

2 boneless skinless chicken breasts, thinly sliced

2 tablespoons avocado oil

¼ cup green onions, sliced

½ cup mushrooms, chopped

¼ green cabbage, thinly sliced

¼ red cabbage, thinly sliced

Butter lettuce for wraps

Carrots, shredded for garnishing

Sprouts, for garnishing

Sesame seeds for topping

Directions

1. In a medium-sized bowl, add sesame oil, balsamic vinegar, coconut aminos, ginger, garlic, salt, pepper, and chicken. Mix thoroughly and set aside.
2. Chop the vegetables accordingly.
3. In a large pan over medium heat, combine avocado oil, onions, and mushrooms. Sauté for about 5 minutes.
4. Add chicken to brown, about 8 minutes.
5. Add cabbage and reduce to low. Cover and let simmer for about 10 minutes, or until cabbage is soft. Stir occasionally.
6. Serve on lettuce and top with carrots, sprouts, and sesame seeds.

Cheesy Chicken and Rice Casserole

Gluten-Free

Serves 6

Ingredients

2 tablespoons butter or avocado oil

2 tablespoons arrowroot starch

2 cups chicken broth

1 cup goat milk

2–3 cups wild rice, cooked

6 medium mushrooms, quartered

4 chicken thighs, chopped

1 shallot, minced

4 sprigs thyme

1½ cups kale, chopped

1 teaspoon garlic, minced

1 teaspoon sea salt

1 teaspoon pepper

1 cup goat cheese, grated

Directions

1. Preheat oven to 350°F.

2. In a small saucepan over medium heat, create roux by whisking butter and arrowroot starch until it bubbles, about 2 minutes.

3. Add broth, whisking continuously to thicken for about 10 minutes.

4. Once the mixture is visibly thicker, add goat milk and continue to whisk for about 5 minutes, allowing to thicken a bit more.

5. Combine all ingredients except for goat cheese in a casserole dish, mixing thoroughly.

6. Top with goat cheese and bake for 40 minutes.

Chicken Parmesan

Gluten-Free

Serves 5

Ingredients

2 tablespoons avocado oil

3–4 eggs, whisked

1 cup cassava root flour

1 cup gluten-free crackers, crushed into fine crumbs

2 cups Pecorino Romano, grated

1 teaspoon smoked paprika

1 teaspoon garlic powder

1 teaspoon dried oregano

1 teaspoon thyme

1 teaspoon sea salt

1 teaspoon pepper

4 boneless, skinless chicken breasts

2–3 cups tomato sauce

4 slices buffalo mozzarella

4 cups zucchini noodles or gluten-free noodles

4 basil leaves for garnish

1 lemon, quartered for topping

Directions

1. Preheat oven to 375°F.

2. In an oven-safe pan over medium heat, warm avocado oil.

3. Meanwhile, place the cassava flour, eggs, and crackers in three separate bowls large enough to dredge the chicken.

4. Add the grated Pecorino, paprika, garlic powder, oregano, thyme, salt, and pepper to the crackers. Mix until well combined.

5. Dredge the chicken breasts one by one on all sides. In this order: cassava, eggs, cracker mixture.

6. With tongs, place dredged chicken breasts into heated oil in the pan.

7. Sauté each side until all the chicken is golden brown but not fully cooked. Remove from heat.

8. To the pan, add the tomato sauce so the chicken breasts are surrounded.

9. Top each chicken breast with mozzarella, and bake in the oven for 40 minutes, or until the internal temperature reaches 165° for each breast.

10. Serve over zucchini noodles, and top with fresh basil and lemon juice.

Blackened Salmon with Creamy Avocado Dressing

Paleo, Gluten-Free

Serves 2

Ingredients

2 tablespoons avocado oil

1 teaspoon garlic powder

1 teaspoon onion powder

1 teaspoon dried oregano

½ teaspoon thyme

½ teaspoon smoked paprika

¼ teaspoon cayenne

1 teaspoon sea salt

1 teaspoon black pepper

4 small salmon filets, about 3–4 ounces each

4 cups massaged kale

1 lime, quartered for garnishing

Dressing

1 avocado

1 clove garlic, peeled

½ jalapeno, chopped

½ cup cilantro, chopped

¼ cup plain goat yogurt

Juice of ½ lime

1 teaspoon lime zest

¼ cup olive oil

¼ teaspoon sea salt

¼ teaspoon pepper

½ teaspoon cumin

Mix the ingredients in a food processor until well combined.

Directions

1. In a large pan over medium heat, warm oil.
2. While pan is heating, combine, garlic powder, onion powder, oregano, thyme, paprika, cayenne, salt, and pepper in a small bowl. Mix until well combined.
3. Coat salmon evenly with seasonings.
4. With tongs, place the salmon filets in the heated oil. Cover and fry each side for about 5–10 minutes, or until the internal temperature reaches 145°F.
5. Serve over massaged kale and top with dressing and lime.

Buddha Bowl with Flank Steak and Cashew Sauce

Paleo

Serves 2–4

Ingredients

1 cup sweet potatoes, chopped

4–5 broccolini stalks

Avocado oil

1 teaspoon sea salt

1 teaspoon pepper

1 tablespoon sesame oil

1 teaspoon sesame seeds

1 teaspoon garlic, minced

½ pound flank steak, thinly sliced

1 cup barley, cooked (or quinoa for gluten-free)

1 cup carrot shavings

½ cup lentils, cooked

1 cup spinach

2–4 eggs, poached

2 tablespoons sprouts

¼ cup red cabbage

Cashew sauce

¼ cup cashew butter

1 tablespoon curry paste

¼ cup full-fat canned coconut milk

4 tablespoons coconut aminos

In a small bowl, combine all cashew sauce ingredients and stir until well combined.

Directions

1. Preheat oven to 400°F.
2. Place sweet potatoes and broccolini on a baking sheet.
3. Coat evenly with avocado oil, salt, and pepper.
4. Bake for 20 minutes.
5. In a pan over medium heat, combine sesame oil, sesame seeds, garlic, and beef.
6. Cook until desired color is achieved, about 8–10 minutes.
7. Layer all ingredients divided evenly between 2–4 bowls for serving.
8. Top with cashew sauce.

Barbecue Slow Cooker Ribs

Paleo, Gluten-Free

Serves 4–6

Ingredients

3 pounds beef ribs

Rub for the ribs

3 tablespoons paprika

1 tablespoon smoked paprika

1 tablespoon garlic powder

1 tablespoon mustard powder

1 tablespoon ground ginger

1 teaspoon salt

¼ teaspoon allspice

¼ teaspoon cayenne pepper

Barbecue Sauce

2 cups organic tomato sauce

½ cup water

½ cup balsamic vinegar

1/3 cup maple syrup

½ tablespoon onion powder

½ tablespoon garlic powder

½ teaspoon sea salt

1 tablespoon stone-ground mustard

¼ cup coconut aminos

Directions

1. Season the ribs with the seasoning blend.
2. Place all barbecue sauce ingredients in a blender and blend until smooth.
3. Pour into a medium saucepan and bring to a boil over medium-high heat.
4. Reduce heat and let simmer for 45 minutes.
5. Place the ribs in the slow cooker on their side (standing up).
6. Pour the desired amount of homemade barbecue sauce over the ribs on both sides.
7. Cook on low for 8 hours, or until fork tender.
8. Add more homemade barbecue sauce if desired.
9. Store extra sauce in the refrigerator.

Creamy Baked Mac and Cheese Casserole

Gluten-Free

Serves 8–10

Ingredients

2 cups brown rice macaroni pasta, cooked

2 cups fresh spinach

2 cups shredded goat cheese, plus extra for topping

½ cup plain goat milk yogurt or plain kefir

1 red bell pepper, chopped

¼ teaspoon onion powder

¼ teaspoon garlic powder

Salt and pepper, to taste

Directions

1. Preheat oven to 350 F.
2. In a bowl combine all the ingredients.
3. Pour mixture into a 9 x 13 greased baking dish.
4. Cover with more goat cheese.
5. Bake for 30 minutes or until top is golden brown.

Slow Cooker Collard Greens with Cajun Spices

Paleo, Gluten-Free

Serves 6–8

Ingredients

8 cups collard greens

8 ounces beef bacon

3 cups chicken bone broth

2 tablespoons Dijon mustard

1 teaspoon garlic powder

¼ teaspoon onion powder

½ teaspoon oregano

½ teaspoon thyme

½ teaspoon smoked paprika

¼ teaspoon cayenne

1 teaspoon salt

1 teaspoon black pepper

Directions

1. Chop collard greens and beef bacon.
2. Add all ingredients to a slow cooker; cook on low for 6–8 hours.

Hasselback Potatoes

Gluten-Free

Serves 10

Ingredients

¼ cup avocado oil

½ cup hazelnuts

2 tablespoons rosemary

1 tablespoon thyme

2 tablespoon garlic, minced

1 teaspoon sea salt

1 teaspoon pepper

5 medium sweet potatoes

¼ cup chives, minced

½ cup maple syrup

¾ cup goat cheese

Directions

1. Preheat oven to 400°F.

2. Combine avocado oil, hazelnuts, rosemary, thyme, garlic, salt and pepper in a food processor and blend until nuts are chunky.

3. Place sweet potatoes in between two spatulas to prevent the potato from moving while cutting.

4. Slice the potato ¾ of the way through, leaving the underside uncut (each cut ½ a centimeter apart).

5. Spread the oil and nut mixture on top of each potato, making sure to get into some of the crevices.

6. In a 9 x 13 baking dish, bake for 1 hour, or until potato is fork tender.

7. Top with chives, maple syrup, and goat cheese.

Cowboy Caviar:
The Best Hearty Salsa Alternative

Vegan, Gluten-Free

Serves 6–8

Ingredients

15 ounces cooked black beans, drained and rinsed

15 ounces black-eyed peas, drained and rinsed

2 Roma tomatoes, diced

1 red bell pepper, diced

1 red onion, diced

1 cup cilantro leaves, chopped

2 tablespoons apple cider vinegar

1 tablespoon maple sugar

½ teaspoon garlic powder

½ teaspoon dried oregano

½ teaspoon dried basil

½ teaspoon chili powder

¼ teaspoon ground black pepper

¼ cup extra virgin olive oil or avocado oil

½ avocado, diced

Tortilla chips for serving

Directions

1. Mix all ingredients together in a large bowl and refrigerate 30 minutes prior to serving.
2. Serve with your favorite grain-free chips or atop your favorite tacos.

Sweet Potato Hash Brown Casserole

Paleo, Gluten-Free

Serves 6–8

Ingredients

1 white onion, chopped

1½ cups goat yogurt

½ cup goat cheddar

½ cup goat feta

2 sweet potatoes, cubed

1–2 tablespoons melted butter

1 teaspoon sea salt

1–2 teaspoons pepper

¼ cup chives, chopped

Directions

1. Preheat oven to 350°F.
2. In medium bowl, mix the onion, yogurt, cheddar, and feta.
3. Add in sweet potatoes and melted butter. Mix until combined.
4. Add mixture to baking dish.
5. Sprinkle extra goat cheddar on top.
6. Add sea salt, pepper, and chives.
7. Bake for 55 minutes.

Queso: The Popular Dip Now Made Healthy

Gluten-Free

Serves 10–12

Ingredients

2 tablespoons grass-fed butter

1 jalapeño, seeds removed and chopped

1 teaspoon sea salt

1 teaspoon pepper

1 teaspoon chili powder

1 teaspoon cumin

1 teaspoon smoked paprika

1 teaspoon garlic

2 tablespoons paleo flour blend

¼ cup plain goat milk yogurt

2 cups full-fat canned coconut cream

3 cups shredded goat cheddar cheese

2–3 Roma tomatoes, diced

Fresh cilantro and avocado for garnish

Directions

1. In a medium saucepan over medium-high heat, melt the butter.

2. Add in jalapeño, stirring until fragrant (about 2 minutes).

3. Add in spices and flour and continue to stir for 2 minutes.

4. Reduce heat to medium and add in yogurt, coconut cream, cheese, and tomatoes, lightly stirring until cheese is completely melted into the mixture.

5. Serve alongside chips in a large bowl, topped with fresh cilantro, avocado, and smoked paprika.

Vegan Mac and Cheese

Vegan, Paleo, Gluten-Free

Serves 6

Ingredients

1 butternut squash, sliced in half lengthwise and seeds discarded

½ white onion, chopped

¼ cup coconut cream

1 teaspoon mustard

1 tablespoon arrowroot powder

1 teaspoon of salt

1 teaspoon of pepper

1 teaspoon of turmeric

1 teaspoon of onion powder

1 teaspoon of garlic powder

1/3–½ cup nutritional yeast

Gluten-free pasta noodles of choice, cooked

Green onions, for garnish

Directions

1. Preheat oven to 400°F.

2. On a baking sheet, lined with parchment paper, place the squash facedown.

3. Bake for 40 minutes, or until fork tender.

4. Scoop the inside of the squash into a high-powdered blender or food processor.

5. Add the remaining ingredients (except the pasta) and blend on high until well combined, adding more herbs and spices as needed.

6. In a large mixing bowl gently stir together the pasta and sauce.

7. Serve topped with green onions.

Summer Sautéed Veggies

Vegan, Paleo, Gluten-Free

Serves 4

Ingredients

1 tablespoon coconut oil

5 cloves garlic, sliced

2 yellow squash, halved and sliced

1 zucchini, halved and sliced

½ teaspoon sea salt

½ teaspoon black pepper

1 cup red grape tomatoes

2 tablespoons chopped fresh oregano

Directions

1. In a large skillet, heat oil over medium-high heat.
2. Add garlic and cook, stirring for about 30 seconds.
3. Add yellow squash, zucchini, salt and pepper. Stir and cook for about 3 minutes.
4. Stir in the tomatoes and continue cooking just until vegetables are tender (about 3 more minutes).
5. Remove from heat and stir in the oregano.

Cauliflower Rice with Cilantro and Lime

Paleo, Gluten-Free

Serves 6–8

Ingredients

2 tablespoons ghee

4 cups grated cauliflower

3 garlic cloves, minced

Juice of one lime

½ cup chopped cilantro

Sea salt and pepper, to taste

Directions

1. In a large pan, melt ghee over medium-high heat.
2. Add in cauliflower and minced garlic, stirring occasionally.
3. Cook cauliflower for 5–10 minutes then remove from heat.
4. In a large mixing bowl, add in cauliflower mixture.
5. Pour in lime juice and mix well.
6. Stir in chopped cilantro.
7. Add sea salt and pepper to taste. Serve immediately.

Gluten-Free Dinner Rolls

Paleo, Gluten-Free

Serves 20

Ingredients

2 cups tapioca starch, plus more for rolling dough

2 cups paleo flour (1 cup almond flour and 1 cup coconut flour)

2 teaspoons Himalayan pink salt

1 cup avocado oil

1 cup warm water

2 eggs, whisked

2 tablespoons grass-fed butter, melted

Directions

1. Heat the oven to 350°F. Line baking sheet with parchment paper.

2. In a large mixing bowl, using a wire whisk or a blending fork, whisk together the tapioca starch, almond flour, coconut flour,and salt. Add in the avocado oil and warm water all at once and continue stirring. Add in the eggs and continue to stir until the mixture becomes doughlike. If the mixture is too soft, add coconut flour one tablespoon at a time until the consistency is correct.

3. Powder your hands with tapioca starch. Scoop out the dough two tablespoons at a time and roll into balls. Place the balls of dough on the prepared baking sheets and bake for 40 minutes or until golden brown.

4. Brush the rolls with melted butter, remove from the pan and allow to cool for 10 minutes before serving.

Baked Vegetable Fries

Vegan, Paleo, Gluten-Free

Serves 2–4

Ingredients

1 cup sliced rutabaga

1 cup sliced carrots

1 cup sliced red bell pepper

1 cup sliced red onion

1 cup sliced portobello mushrooms

Ghee or coconut oil

2–4 teaspoons sea salt

2 teaspoons black pepper

2 teaspoons onion powder

2 teaspoons garlic powder

Directions

1. Preheat oven to 425°F.
2. Cut vegetables into thin long strips.
3. Toss in a bowl with ghee or melted coconut oil. Sprinkle with sea salt, black pepper, onion powder, and garlic powder.
4. Place on a baking sheet with parchment paper and bake for 40 minutes.
5. Dip in sauce of your choosing such as honey mustard.

Soft, Chewy Chocolate Chip Cookies

Paleo, Gluten-Free

Makes 8–10 cookies

Ingredients

¼ cup coconut oil, melted

1/3 cup coconut sugar

1 egg

2 tablespoons almond butter

1 teaspoon vanilla extract

½ teaspoon Himalayan pink salt

1 teaspoon baking powder

1 tablespoon arrowroot starch

½ cup + 1 tablespoon Paleo flour (grain-free flour such as cassava or coconut)

½ cup dark chocolate chips (70 percent or darker)

Directions

1. Preheat oven to 350°F.

2. In a medium bowl, whisk together the coconut oil, coconut sugar, egg, almond butter, and vanilla extract. Set aside.

3. In a small bowl, add in the remaining dry ingredients, except the chocolate chips, and mix until well combined.

4. Add the dry ingredients to the wet ingredients, mixing until well incorporated, then fold in the chocolate chips.

5. Cover dough and let chill in the fridge for about 10 minutes to make it easier to work with (optional).

6. Scoop out about 2 tablespoons of dough and form into a cookie shape. Place each cookie on a 9 x 11 baking sheet, spaced 1–2 inches apart.

7. Bake for 10–11 minutes.

Key Lime Pie

Paleo, Gluten-Free

Serves 8–10

Ingredients

1 tablespoon coconut oil

2 tablespoons arrowroot starch

2 cups evaporated or condensed coconut milk

½ cup lime juice

1 teaspoon lime zest

1 teaspoon vanilla extract

½ cup maple syrup

½ teaspoon sea salt

1 gluten-free pie crust (store-bought or homemade)

2–3 limes, sliced for garnishing

Directions

1. In a saucepan over medium heat, combine starch and coconut oil. Whisk to create a roux.

2. After about one minute, add coconut milk. Whisk continuously until mixture thickens into a custard-like consistency, about 10 minutes.

3. Add lime juice, lime zest, vanilla, maple syrup, and salt. Whisk until mixture thickens even more, about 5 minutes.

4. Pour mixture into pie crust and allow to cool, then chill the rest of the way in the freezer, about one hour.

5. Top with sliced lime for garnish and serve.

White Chocolate: A Paleo and Vegan Candy

Vegan, Paleo, Gluten-Free

Servings: 30–40 candies

Ingredients

1 cup cashews

1 pound raw cacao butter

2 tablespoons powdered coconut milk

½ cup maple syrup

1 vanilla bean, cut and scraped

Directions

1. Soak cashews for at least 1 hour.
2. Drain cashews and blend them in a food processor until smooth.
3. In a double boiler, melt cacao butter, and add cashews, coconut milk, syrup, and vanilla bean.
4. Stir until well combined and then pour into a mold of desired shape.
5. Allow to cool and then chill in freezer until solidified, about 1 hour.

Chocolate Chip Pizookie with Butterscotch Drizzle

Gluten-Free

Serves 8–10

Ingredients

Pizookie

¾ cup coconut oil, solid at room temperature

½ cup coconut sugar

2 eggs

1 teaspoon vanilla extract

½ teaspoon baking soda

½ teaspoon sea salt

¼ cup cocoa or cacao powder

2 cups Paleo flour (grain-free flour such as cassava or coconut)

½ cup dark chocolate chips (70 percent or darker)

½ cup hazelnuts, chopped

Butterscotch Drizzle

½ cup coconut sugar

¼ cup coconut butter

½ cup coconut cream

1 teaspoon sea salt

1 teaspoon vanilla

Directions

1. Preheat oven to 350 degrees F.
2. In a medium-sized bowl, combine ½ cup coconut sugar, coconut oil, 1 teaspoon vanilla and eggs, mixing until well combined.
3. Add flour, baking soda, cacao powder and ½ teaspoon salt, mixing until well combined.
4. Add chocolate chips and hazelnuts and mix thoroughly.
5. Spread dough evenly into a greased circular pan.
6. Bake for 12–15 minutes.
7. In a small saucepan over medium heat, combine remaining coconut sugar and coconut butter, whisking constantly to prevent burning.
8. When mixture resembles a caramel paste (after about 5–8 minutes), bring temperature to medium-low.
9. Add coconut cream, remaining vanilla and sea salt.
10. Bring to a boil on medium heat, continuously whisking.
11. When mixture is thick like butterscotch (after about 8 minutes), remove from heat.
12. Serve pizookie topped with butterscotch sauce.

Cinnamon Rolls with Cream Cheese Icing

Gluten-Free

Makes 7–9 rolls

Ingredients

Dough

½ cup warm goat milk

1 package active dry yeast

2 cups cassava flour

½ cup tapioca starch

1 cup boiled sweet potato, mashed

¼ cup coconut sugar

4 tablespoons grass-fed butter

1 egg

½ teaspoon salt

Filling

1 cup coconut sugar

4 tablespoons grass-fed butter

2 tablespoons cinnamon

¼ teaspoon cardamom

Icing

4 ounces raw cream cheese

4 tablespoons grass-fed butter

½ cup coconut sugar

1 tablespoon vanilla extract

2 teaspoons orange zest

Directions

1. Preheat oven to 350°F. Grease a medium-sized baking dish.
2. In a large bowl, mix warm goat milk and yeast. Rest for 10 minutes. If yeast clumps, start again.
3. Add dough ingredients: cassava, tapioca, sweet potato, sugar, butter, egg, and salt. Mix until mostly combined and then knead with hands into a ball. Cover and rest dough for 1 hour.
4. In a small bowl, mix filling ingredients. Set aside
5. With parchment on a flat surface, roll dough into a large rectangle about ¼ inch thick.
6. With your hand, spread the filling evenly on top of the flattened dough.
7. With the help of the parchment paper, carefully roll the dough into itself. Roll this as tight as possible.
8. Using a string, tie one knot around the cinnamon roll. Pull both sides of the string to carefully cut the cinnamon roll. Repeat until all rolls are cut.
9. Place each roll into the greased baking dish.
10. Bake for 15–20 minutes.
11. In a separate small bowl, mix icing ingredients.
12. Spread icing on cinnamon rolls and serve.

Vegan, Paleo Apple Fritters

Vegan, Paleo, Gluten-Free

Makes 7–9 fritters

Ingredients

Batter

2 Granny Smith apples, chopped

1 tablespoon coconut oil

1 cup pecans, chopped

4 tablespoons coconut sugar (optional)

2 cups Paleo flour (grain-free flour such as cassava or coconut)

2 teaspoons baking powder

4 tablespoons maple syrup

4 tablespoons flax meal

2/3 cup water

1 cup almond milk

2 tablespoons pumpkin pie spice

Glaze (optional)

1/3 cup maple or coconut sugar

1/3 cup coconut butter

2 tablespoons water

Directions

1. Preheat oven to 350°F degrees.

2. In a large pan, on medium, fry apples, coconut oil, pecans, and coconut sugar for about 10 minutes or until soft. Set aside to cool.

3. In a large bowl, mix flour, baking powder, maple syrup, flax meal, water, almond milk, pumpkin pie spice and apple mixture.

4. Scoop batter (about 1/3 cup) onto a lined baking sheet, creating the fritter. Repeat until you run out of batter.

5. Bake for 15–20 minutes.

6. In a small saucepan, on medium, combine glaze ingredients.

7. Stir often until the glaze becomes thick but runny.

8. Top fritters with the glaze and serve.

Churros: The Popular Spanish Snack

Paleo, Gluten-Free

Serves 6

Ingredients

1 cup water

1/3 cup butter

2 tablespoon maple sugar

2 cups Paleo flour blend

1 teaspoon vanilla extract

2 eggs

½ teaspoon cinnamon

¼ teaspoon sea salt

Cinnamon and maple sugar, for topping

Directions

1. Preheat oven to 350°F.
2. In a saucepan over medium heat, melt butter and maple sugar in water, bringing it to a boil.
3. Remove from heat and stir in flour.
4. Add in vanilla and eggs, stirring until well combined.
5. Transfer mixture to a piping bag.
6. On a baking sheet lined with parchment paper, use the piping bag to add 4-inch strips of the churro mixture to the pan.
7. Bake for 15–20 minutes.
8. Sprinkle or roll each churro in the cinnamon and maple sugar mixture.

Paleo Brownies with 8 Perfect Ingredients

Paleo, Gluten-Free

Serves 12

Ingredients

½ cup coconut oil

1/3 cup dark chocolate chips

2 eggs

½–¾ cup maple sugar

¾ teaspoon Himalayan pink salt

3 tablespoons arrowroot starch

¼–½ cup cocoa or cacao powder

2 teaspoons vanilla

Directions

1. Preheat oven to 350°F.
2. Melt the coconut oil and chocolate chips in a small pot over medium heat.
3. Using a hand mixer, mix all the other ingredients together in a large bowl until the batter is thick.
4. Pour contents into an 8.5" x 4.5" x 2.75" loaf pan.
5. Bake for 30 minutes.
6. Allow to cool for 15 minutes.

Gluten-Free Apple Galette

Gluten-Free

Serves 6

Ingredients

2–3 apples of choice, thinly sliced

Flour Mixture

1/3 cup sprouted almonds

2 tablespoons gluten-free sprouted flour blend (brown rice, oat, sorghum)

5 tablespoons maple sugar, divided

Galette Crust

2½ cups gluten-free sprouted flour blend (brown rice, oat, sorghum)

1 teaspoon Himalayan salt

1 tablespoon maple sugar

2 sticks unsalted grass-fed butter, chilled and cubed

¼ cup ice water

Coconut cream

Directions

1. Process the flour mixture and set aside.
2. Process the first three ingredients of the galette crust mixture.
3. Add in the butter, while pulsing until well combined.
4. Add in ice water, little by little, while pulsing until thick dough is formed.
5. Roll dough into a disc and wrap with plastic wrap.
6. Refrigerate for 2 hours.
7. Preheat oven to 400°F.
8. Remove the galette crust and roll dough into a 10–12-inch circle.
9. Coat with some of the flour mixture.
10. Pile the apples onto the dough, slightly mounding it in the center and leaving a 2-inch border around the edge. Fold the rim of the dough up and over the edge of the apple filling, overlapping the dough as you go around and pleating the dough.
11. Brush with coconut cream and sprinkle with more maple sugar.
12. Refrigerate for 25 minutes.
13. Bake for 50 minutes to 1 hour, or until crust is golden.

Watermelon Pizza

Vegan, Paleo, Gluten-Free

Serves 2–3

Ingredients

1 watermelon, sliced

Coconut yogurt

3 kiwi, chopped

1 mango, chopped

1 pineapple, chopped

1 package strawberries, blueberries, raspberries all sliced

10 cherries, pitted and sliced

Raw honey and mint leaves for topping

Directions

1. Cut the slices of watermelon into four pieces.

2. Top with yogurt, fresh fruit, and mint.

3. Drizzle with raw honey. Serve.

Thai Iced Tea

Vegan, Paleo, Gluten-Free

Serves 2

Ingredients

1 cup boiled water

4 cloves, whole

½ teaspoon vanilla extract

1 teaspoon cardamom

2 star anise

2 organic black tea bags

2 organic orange blossom tea bags or 1 teaspoon orange zest

½ cup cold water

¼ cup coconut milk

1 tablespoon maple syrup (optional)

Directions

1. In a large cup with a slanted edge for pouring, combine all ingredients except for the cold water and coconut milk.

2. Stir ingredients and steep tea for 8–10 minutes.

3. Add ½ cup of cold water.

4. Fill two tall glasses to the brim with ice.

5. Using a small mesh strainer, pour tea evenly between two glasses.

6. Top each glass with coconut milk, stir, and serve.

Hydrating Watermelon Smoothie with Strawberries and Banana

Vegan, Paleo, Gluten-Free

Serves 2

Ingredients

1 banana

2 cups fresh or frozen seedless watermelon

½ cup frozen strawberries

1 cup plain coconut milk yogurt

1 tablespoon chia seeds (optional)

Maple syrup to taste (optional)

Directions

Add all the ingredients to a blender, blending until well combined.

Strawberry Banana Smoothie

Vegan, Paleo, Gluten-Free

Serves 1

Ingredients

1 cup strawberries

½ banana

½ cup coconut milk

½ cup ice

½ scoop vanilla protein powder

Stevia to taste

Directions

Add all ingredients to blender and blend until well combined.

Bone Broth Protein Mocha Fudge Smoothie

Paleo, Gluten-Free

Serves 1–2

Ingredients

1 cup frozen banana

¼ cup raw cashews

2 tablespoons cocoa powder

1 teaspoon carob powder

1 teaspoon instant coffee

12 ounces coconut milk

1 teaspoon raw honey

1 scoop of protein powder made from bone broth (vanilla or chocolate)

Directions

Place all ingredients in blender and purée until smooth, adding water and ice to blend as necessary.

Gut-Healing Smoothie

Paleo, Gluten-Free

Serves 4

Ingredients

1–2 cups full-fat coconut milk or almond milk

2 cups kale

2 cups spinach

½ avocado

2 frozen bananas, cut into chunks

1 teaspoon freshly grated ginger

½ tablespoon chia or flax seeds

½ tablespoon bee pollen

1 tablespoon hemp hearts

1 tablespoon raw honey or manuka honey

2 tablespoons collagen protein or whey protein

Directions

1. Place all ingredients in a blender and blend on high until smooth (about 2–3 minutes).
2. Serve over ice.

Omega Blueberry Smoothie

Gluten-Free

Serves 1

Ingredients

1 cup blueberries

¼ cup coconut milk

1 tablespoon sprouted flax meal

1 scoop vanilla whey protein powder

Directions

Add all ingredients to a blender and blend until smooth.

Orange Carrot Ginger Juice – Kid's Favorite

Vegan, Paleo, Gluten-Free

Serves 2

Ingredients

6 carrots

1 orange

1 knob ginger

1 cucumber

Directions

1. Add all ingredients to vegetable juicer.
2. Gently stir juice and consume immediately.

Strawberry Lemonade

Paleo, Gluten-Free

Serves 2–4

Ingredients

3 cups of spring or filtered water

½ cup organic lemon juice

2 cups organic strawberries, fresh or frozen

Raw local honey, to taste

Directions

Combine all ingredients in a blender until smooth.

Peachy Super Kale Shake

Vegan, Paleo, Gluten-Free

Serves 2

Ingredients

1 cup baby kale leaves

½ cup frozen pineapple

½ cup frozen strawberries

½ cup fresh diced peaches

1 cup canned coconut milk or water

Directions

1. In a high-speed blender, add ingredients and puree on high.
2. Serve and enjoy immediately.

Chocolate Banana Nut Smoothie

Vegan, Paleo, Gluten-Free

Serves 1

Ingredients

1 cup coconut milk

1/3 cup sprouted almond butter

1 banana, peeled

2 tablespoons cacao powder

2 cups ice cubes

Stevia to taste (optional)

Directions

Place all ingredients in a blender and blend until smooth.

Miso Soup with Mushrooms

Vegan, Gluten-Free

Serves 2

Ingredients

4 cups organic broth or water

2 tablespoons mellow white miso

2 cups fresh mushrooms or ½ cup dried, chopped

1 large yellow or red onion, diced

2 cloves garlic, pressed or minced

1–2 teaspoons grated ginger

2 cups coarsely chopped collard greens

2 tablespoons coconut aminos

Directions

1. In a medium pot, heat broth or water over medium-high heat. Once simmering, remove about half a cup and whisk together with the miso, incorporating until smooth.

2. Add the miso mixture back to the pot along with the mushrooms, onion, garlic, ginger, collards, and coconut aminos.

3. Return to a simmer and decrease heat to low, simmering gently for 20 minutes.

Chicken Bone Broth

Paleo, Gluten-Free

Serving size varies

Ingredients

4 pounds chicken necks/feet/wings

3 carrots, chopped

3 celery stalks, chopped

2 medium onions, peel on, sliced in half lengthwise and quartered

4 garlic cloves, peel on and smashed

1 teaspoon Himalayan salt

1 teaspoon whole peppercorns

3 tablespoons apple cider vinegar

2 bay leaves

3 sprigs fresh thyme

5–6 sprigs parsley

1 teaspoon oregano

18–20 cups cold water

Directions

1. Place all ingredients in a 10-quart capacity slow cooker.
2. Simmer for 24–48 hours, skimming fat occasionally.
3. Remove from heat and allow to cool slightly.
4. Discard solids and strain remainder in a bowl through a colander.
5. Let stock cool to room temperature, cover, and chill.
6. Use within a week or freeze up to three months.

Beef Bone Broth

Paleo, Gluten-Free

Serving size varies

Ingredients

4 pounds beef bones with marrow

4 carrots, chopped

4 celery stalks, chopped

2 medium onions, peel on, sliced in half lengthwise and quartered

4 garlic cloves, peel on and smashed

1 teaspoon kosher salt

1 teaspoon whole peppercorns

2 bay leaves

3 sprigs fresh thyme

5–6 sprigs parsley

¼ cup apple cider vinegar

18–20 cups cold water

Directions

1. Place all ingredients in a 10-quart capacity slow cooker.
2. Simmer for 24–48 hours, occasionally skimming the fat that rises to the surface.
3. Remove from heat and allow to cool slightly.
4. Discard solids and strain remainder in a bowl through a colander.
5. Let stock cool to room temperature, cover, and chill.
6. Use within a week or freeze up to 3 months.

Potato Leek Soup

Gluten-Free

Serves 10–12

Ingredients

2 medium heads of cauliflower

½ cup unsalted grass-fed butter

1 small red onion, diced

1 small yellow onion, diced

2 leeks, sliced

3 stalks of celery, chopped

2 medium Yukon potatoes, peeled and diced

1 bay leaf

3 sprigs fresh thyme

1 32-ounce container of chicken broth

2 cups vegetable broth

1 package turkey bacon, small diced

Salt and pepper to taste

Sliced green onions

Directions

1. Chop cauliflower then add to a food processor and pulse until rice-like consistency. Set aside.

2. In a large saucepan over medium heat, melt the butter. Add in the onions, leeks, and celery. Cover and cook for 10 minutes.

3. Stir in the potato, bay leaf, and thyme. Cook for 10 minutes.

4. Add the broth, cauliflower, and turkey bacon, bringing mixture to a boil.

5. Reduce heat and simmer for 30 minutes.

6. Remove from heat. Carefully remove the bay leaf and thyme.

7. Use an immersion hand blender to puree the soup in the pot (or puree in a high-speed blender). Allow soup to rest for 5 minutes. Add salt and pepper to taste.

8. Top with sliced green onions.

Tuscan White Bean Soup

Vegan, Gluten-Free

Serves 6–8

Ingredients

2 tablespoons avocado oil

1 white onion, chopped

3 carrots, diced

3 stalks of celery, chopped

3 cloves garlic, minced

1 zucchini, diced

1 yellow squash, diced

6 cups vegetable broth or chicken broth

1 tablespoon sage leaves

½ cup fresh parsley

1 Roma tomato, diced

1½ cups purple cabbage, sliced

1½ cups lacinato kale

2 15.5-ounce cans of cannellini beans, rinsed

Salt and pepper to taste

Crumbled goat cheese for topping (optional)

Directions

1. In a stockpot add avocado oil and panfry the onions, carrots, celery, garlic, and squash over medium heat.
2. Add broth.
3. Add in the rest of the ingredients and simmer for 30 minutes.
4. Top with crumbled goat cheese (optional).

Chicken Vegetable Soup

Paleo, Gluten-Free

Serves 4–5

Ingredients

3 organic chicken breasts, diced

3–4 carrots, chopped

1 onion, chopped

3–4 celery stalks, chopped

1 zucchini, thinly sliced

5 cups chicken broth

Sea salt and black pepper to taste

2 ounces raw cheese

Directions

1. Place the chicken and vegetables in a large soup pot and cover with cold water. Heat and simmer, uncovered, until chicken is thoroughly cooked (usually over 30 minutes).

2. Strain the chicken and vegetables, then add them back into the pot.

3. Pour in the broth, season with sea salt and black pepper, and heat up for 10 minutes.

4. Top with cheese and serve.

Black Bean Soup

Vegan, Gluten-Free

Serves 4

Ingredients

2 15-ounce cans organic black beans

1 cup water

2 tablespoons coconut oil

¼ cup chopped white onion

¼ cup chopped green onions

¼ cup chopped red bell pepper

¼ cup chopped mushrooms

3 minced garlic cloves

1 teaspoon sea salt

1 teaspoon chili powder

1 teaspoon cumin

Hot sauce, to taste (optional)

Directions

1. In a food processor or blender, blend one can of black beans with one cup of water until smooth.
2. In a medium saucepan, add in coconut oil over medium-high heat.
3. Sauté onions, pepper, mushrooms, and garlic until tender.
4. Add black bean mixture from the blender and stir on medium-low heat.
5. Add in second can of beans and continue cooking 5–10 minutes.
6. Add sea salt, chili powder, cumin, and hot sauce to taste.
7. Serve hot.

Taco Soup

Gluten-Free

Serves 8–10

Ingredients

2 pounds ground bison

2 cups onions, diced

2 cans of choice black and kidney beans

2 cups organic corn

1 14-ounce can of organic plum tomatoes

5 tomatoes, diced

1 14-ounce can of tomatoes with chilis

2 tablespoons cumin

1 tablespoon chili powder

1 tablespoon garlic powder

Salt to taste

Peppers, sliced

Directions

1. Brown the ground bison in a medium-high heated skillet. (Remember: The ground bison will continue to cook in the slow cooker, so it doesn't have to be overcooked.)

2. Place browned bison and all the other ingredients into a slow cooker and gently mix with a wooden spoon.

3. Cook on low for 8–10 hours.

4. Serve in soup bowls placed on plate, with sliced peppers on the side.

5. Top with your favorite toppings, such as avocado, diced green onion, and shredded raw cheese.

Creamy Broccoli Soup with Cheese

Paleo, Gluten-Free

Serves 4

Ingredients

¼ cup ghee

1 cup green onions

6 garlic cloves, minced

6 cups baby kale

8 cups chopped broccoli florets

32 ounces chicken or vegetable broth

16 ounces kefir

2 cups raw cheddar cheese

Directions

1. Place the ghee, green onions, garlic, kale, and broccoli in a large pot and sauté them for 10 minutes over medium-high heat, stirring consistently.
2. Add in the chicken or vegetable broth and heat for another 5–10 minutes.
3. Pour the mixture into a blender and blend until smooth.
4. Pour contents back into the pot and simmer over high heat for 10 minutes.
5. Add the kefir and cheese and stir well.
6. Serve immediately.

Cold Melon Berry Soup

Vegan, Paleo, Gluten-Free

Serves 4

Ingredients

3 medium cantaloupes

¼ cup fresh lemon or lime juice

½ cup fresh blueberries

½ cup fresh strawberry

Directions

1. Remove the peel and slice the melon into large chunks.
2. Puree melon in a blender or food processor until it has liquified.
3. Gently mix in lemon or lime juice and chill the mixture in the freezer for 20–30 minutes.
4. Serve in individual bowls, garnished with fresh berries.

Vegan Granola

Serves 2-4

Ingredients

1 cup crushed almonds

1 cup oats

1 cup sunflower seeds

1 cup pumpkin seeds

½ cup coconut flakes

1 cup honey

1 teaspoon cinnamon

Directions

1. Preheat oven to 250°F.
2. Mix all ingredients and spread out on a nonstick cookie sheet.
3. Bake for 20 minutes.
4. Stir and continue to bake another 20 minutes, stirring periodically to prevent burning. The granola should be lightly browned.
5. Remove from oven and serve warm or cool thoroughly and store in tightly sealed container or plastic bags.
6. Option: After the granola is cooled, add raisins or other organic, unsulphured dehydrated fruit.

Black Bean Soup

Serves 2-4

Ingredients

1 pound of black beans, soaked overnight, rinsed, and drained

8 cups vegetable stock

1 whole onion

2 bay leaves

2 garlic cloves, minced

1 tablespoon olive oil

1 cup celery, chopped

1 potato, grated

1 yellow or red pepper, chopped

1 cup carrots, grated

2 tablespoons cilantro

1 tablespoon parsley

2 tablespoons marjoram

1 teaspoon honey

Sea salt, to taste

Directions

1. Place beans in pot with vegetable stock, whole onion, and bay leaves.
2. Cook 2½ hours or until beans are tender.
3. Remove onion and bay leaves; chop onion.
4. Sauté garlic in a tablespoon of olive oil until tender.
5. During last hour of cooking, add vegetables and seasonings to beans.
6. Bring to a boil, lower heat to simmer, and cook until veggies and beans are tender.

Minestrone Soup

Serves 2-4

Ingredients

1½ cups dried garbanzo beans

2 cups dried red kidney beans

½ cup carrots, chopped

½ cup onion, chopped

½ cup celery, chopped

1 clove garlic, minced

3 medium tomatoes (or 1 14-ounce can of unsweetened, unsalted Italian tomatoes), peeled and diced

¼ teaspoon oregano

¾ teaspoon basil

¼ teaspoon thyme

1 cup cabbage, chopped

½ cup fresh parsley, minced

1 package spinach noodles, cooked

8 cups vegetable stock

Sea salt, to taste

Directions

1. Soak garbanzo and kidney beans overnight, drain and rinse.
2. Cook garbanzo and kidney beans as per directions on package; drain.
3. In a large pot sauté carrots, onion, celery, cabbage, and garlic in water or soup stock over medium heat for 5–7 minutes.
4. Stir in beans, tomatoes, oregano, basil, and thyme.
5. Bring to a boil, then turn heat down and simmer 10 minutes.
6. Stir in cabbage and parsley with lid partially on for about 15 minutes or until cabbage is tender.
7. Add more soup stock or tomatoes as needed.
8. Serve over spinach noodles.

Stir-Fry Vegetables

Serves 2-4

Ingredients

1–2 tablespoons olive oil

1 red onion, sliced

3 stalks celery, thinly sliced

½ cup broccoli, chopped

1 bell pepper, sliced

3 carrots, peeled and sliced

½ cup cauliflower, chopped

1 cup zucchini, thinly sliced

1 cup yellow squash, thinly sliced

1 teaspoon sea salt

1 tablespoon Asian seasoning (or a mix of garlic powder, onion powder, ginger powder, and black pepper)

Directions

1. Stir-fry all vegetables in olive oil until tender.

2. Add salt and seasoning.

3. Serve alone or over brown rice.

The Green Beastie Smoothie

Vegan, Gluten-Free

Serves 1

Ingredients

1½ cups spinach

1 cup mango

1 cup avocado

1 teaspoon cocoa powder

1 teaspoon spirulina

½ cup water

Handful of ice

Directions

Place ingredients into a high-powered blender and mix.

Harira

Serves 4

Note: Harira is a great recipe for the Daniel Fast as it has nearly 15 grams of protein per serving.

Ingredients

2 tablespoons healthy oil, such as coconut oil or olive oil

1 cup chopped onion

½ cup chopped celery

2 cups warm water

Pinch of saffron threads

½ teaspoon salt, divided

¼ teaspoon peeled fresh ginger, minced

¼ teaspoon ground red pepper

¼ teaspoon ground cinnamon

2 garlic cloves, minced

2 cups organic mushroom broth

1½ cups chopped and seeded plum tomatoes

½ cup dried small red lentils

2 15-ounce cans no-salt-added chickpeas, drained

3 tablespoons chopped fresh cilantro

3 tablespoons chopped fresh parsley

Directions

1. Heat oil in a large saucepan on medium heat.
2. Add onion and celery and sauté 4 minutes or until tender.
3. Combine warm water and saffron; let stand 2 minutes.
4. Add ¼ teaspoon salt, ginger, red pepper, cinnamon, and garlic.
5. Cook 1 minute. Add saffron water mixture, broth, tomatoes, lentils, and chickpeas.
6. Bring to boil; then reduce heat.
7. Simmer 20 minutes or until lentils are tender.
8. Stir in cilantro, parsley, and remaining ¼ teaspoon salt.

Lebanese Fattoush Salad

Vegan, Gluten-Free

Serves 4

Ingredients

4 cups romaine, chopped

¼ cup white onions, chopped

1 cucumber, sliced

½ cup cherry tomatoes, sliced

4–5 mint leaves, chopped

4–5 basil leaves, chopped

¼ green onions, chopped

Dressing

¼ cup extra virgin olive oil

Juice of ½ lemon

½ teaspoon garlic powder

¼ teaspoon salt

1 teaspoon ground sumac

Directions

1. Mix all the ingredients for the dressing and set aside.
2. In a large bowl, mix together the salad ingredients.
3. Drizzle the dressing over the salad and mix until well combined.

Cucumber Salad with Tomato and Onion

Vegan, Paleo, Gluten-Free

Serves 4–6

Ingredients

1 cucumber, quartered

12 Kumato tomatoes, sliced in half

½ red onion, chopped

2–3 green onions, chopped

8 basil leaves, chiffonade

Dressing

2–3 tablespoons apple cider vinegar

2–3 tablespoons olive oil

¼ teaspoon Himalayan pink salt

¼ teaspoon pepper

Directions

1. Mix the dressing together in a small bowl and set aside.
2. In a medium bowl, mix together the salad ingredients.
3. Drizzle on the dressing, mix together thoroughly and serve.

Quinoa Salad with Fruit

Vegan, Gluten-Free

Serves 4

Ingredients

1 cup quinoa

¼ cup raw honey or maple syrup

Juice of 1 lime

1 cup blueberries

1 cup strawberries, chopped

1 cup mango, chopped

1 cup honeydew, chopped

1/3 cup basil, chiffonade

Directions

1. Cook quinoa according to package.
2. In a small mixing bowl, whisk the honey or syrup and lime until well combined and set aside.
3. In a large bowl, add cooked quinoa, fruit, basil and mix until well incorporated.
4. Add honey lime mixture, stirring until evenly mixed.
5. Serve and enjoy!

Cauliflower Tabbouleh Salad

Vegan, Paleo, Gluten-Free

Serves 6

Ingredients

1 large head cauliflower, chopped

½ cup lemon juice

¾ cup extra virgin olive oil

1 bunch parsley, chopped

1 bunch green onions, chopped

2 cups Roma tomatoes, chopped

1 teaspoon salt

1 teaspoon pepper

Directions

1. Put cauliflower in a food processor and pulse until rice-like consistency.
2. In a large bowl, combine the cauliflower and the lemon juice.
3. Add the olive oil, parsley, green onions, tomatoes, salt, and pepper.
4. Stir well.
5. Taste and add more salt and pepper if needed.
6. Cover and refrigerate for at least 4 hours, stirring once each hour.

Garden Squash with Sun-Dried Tomatoes

Vegan, Paleo, Gluten-Free

Serves 6

Ingredients

1–2 tablespoons olive oil

2 shallots, finely diced

4 medium-sized yellow squash, ¼-inch slices

4 medium-sized zucchini, ¼-inch slices

1 6-ounce jar sun-dried tomatoes, undrained

2 tablespoons fresh basil, sliced thin

Sea salt and black pepper to taste

Directions

1. In a medium skillet, add oil, shallots, and both squashes. Sauté until squash is becoming soft and lightly browned over medium-high heat.

2. Add sun-dried tomatoes and basil.

3. Toss gently to mix.

4. Serve immediately.

NOTES

Part 1: FASTING IS NOT A FAD

1. Selene Yeager, *The Doctors Book of Food Remedies: The Latest Findings on the Power of Food to Treat and Prevent Health Problems—From Aging and Diabetes to Ulcers and Yeast Infections* (New York: Rodale Inc., 2007).

2. "Fasting Quotes," All About Fasting, accessed June 7, 2020, https://www.allaboutfasting.com/fasting-quotes.html.

3. "Fasting Quotes," All About Fasting.

4. "Fasting," Encyclopedia.com, updated May 14, 2020, https://www.encyclopedia.com/philosophy-and-religion/other-religious-beliefs-and-general-terms/religion-general/fasting.

5. "Fasting Quotes," All About Fasting.

Part 2: FASTING FUNDAMENTALS

1. Nick English, "Autophagy: The Real Way to Cleanse Your Body," *Atlanta Journal-Constitution*, February 29, 2016, https://www.ajc.com/lifestyles/health/autophagy-the-real-way-cleanse-your-body/06qE9DQ4oT2hJ5hMNM1NpM/.

2. Congcong He, Michael C. Bassik, Viviana Moresi, Kai Sun, Yongjie Wei, Zhongju Zou, Zhenyi An et al., "Exercise-induced BCL2-regulated Autophagy Is Required for Muscle Glucose Homeostasis," *Nature* 481, no. 7382 (January 18, 2012): 511–515.

3. English, "Autophagy: The Real Way to Cleanse Your Body"

4. Bérengère Coupé, Yuko Ishii, Marcelo O. Dietrich, Masaaki Komatsu, Tamas L. Horvath, and Sebastien G. Bouret, "Loss of Autophagy in Pro-Opiomelanocortin Neurons Perturbs Axon Growth and Causes Metabolic Dysregulation," *Cell Metabolism* 15, no. 2 (January 26, 2012): 247–255.

5. Adam Freund, Arturo V. Orjalo, Pierre-Yves Desprez, and Judith Campisi, "Inflammatory Networks during Cellular Senescence: Causes and Consequences," *Trends in Molecular Medicine* 16, no. 5 (May 2010): 238–246.

6. C. Ntsapi and B. Loos, "Caloric Restriction and the Precision-Control of Autophagy: A Strategy for Delaying Neurodegenerative Disease Progression," *Experimental Gerontology* 83 (October 20016): 97–111.

7. Congcong He, Rhea Sumpter, and Beth Levine, "Exercise Induces Autophagy in Peripheral Tissues and in the Brain," *Autophagy* 8, no. 10 (October 2012): 1548–1551.

8. Stephen D. Anton, Keelin Moehl, William T. Donahoo, Krisztina Marosi, Stephanie Lee, Arch G. Mainous, III, Christiaan Leeuwenburgh, and Mark P. Mattson, "Flipping the Metabolic Switch: Understanding and Applying Health Benefits of Fasting," *Obesity* 26, no. 2 (February 2018): 254–268.

9. Valter D. Longo and Satchidananda Panda, "Fasting, Circadian Rhythms, and Time-Restricted Feeding in Healthy Lifespan," *Cell Metabolism* 23, no. 6 (June 14, 2016): 1048–1059.

10. Michael J. Wilkinson, Emily N.C. Manoogian, Adena Zadourian, Hannah Lo, Savannah Fakhouri, Azarin Shoghi, Xinran Wang et al., "Ten-Hour Time-Restricted Eating Reduces Weight, Blood Pressure, and Atherogenic Lipids in Patients with Metabolic Syndrome," *Cell Metabolism* 31, no. 1 (January 7, 2020): 92–104.

11. Chaix, A., Zarrinpar, A., Miu, P., & Panda, S., "Time-restricted feeding is a preventative and therapeutic intervention against diverse nutritional challenges," *Cell Metabolism 20, no. 6 (June 2014)*: 991–1005. https://doi.org/10.1016/j.cmet.2014.11.001

12. Saeid Golbid, Andreas Daiber, Bato Korac, Huige Li, M. Faadiel Essop, and Ismail Laher, "Health Benefits of Fasting and Caloric Restriction," *Current Diabetes Reports* 17, no. 12 (October 23, 2017): 123.

13. Suriani Ismail, Rosliza Abdul Manaf, and Aidalina Mahmud, "Comparison of Time-Restricted Feeding and Islamic Fasting: A Scoping Review," *Eastern Mediterranean Health Journal* 25, no. 4 (June 2019): 239–245.

14. Lisa S. Chow, Emily N. C. Manoogian, Alison Alvear, Jason G. Fleischer, Honoree Thor, Katrina Dietsche, Qi Wang et al., "Time-Restricted Eating Effects on Body Composition and Metabolic Measures in Humans who are Overweight: A Feasibility Study," *Obesity* 28, no. 5 (May 2020): 860–869.

15. Tatiana Moro, Grant Tinsley, Antonino Bianco, Giuseppe Marcolin, Quirico Francesco Pacelli, Giuseppe Battaglia, Antonio Palma et al., "Effects of eight weeks of time-restricted feeding (16/8) on basal metabolism, maximal strength, body composition, inflammation, and cardiovascular risk factors in resistance-trained males," *Journal of Translational Medicine* 14, no. 1 (October 13, 2016): 290.

PART 3: THE WHY BEHIND FASTING

1. "Obesity and Overweight," U.S. Department of Health & Human Services, accessed June 8, 2020, https://www.cdc.gov/nchs/fastats/obesity-overweight.htm.

2. John LaRosa, "Top 9 Things to Know About the Weight Loss Industry," Marketresearch.com, March 6, 2019, https://blog.marketresearch.com/u.s.-weight-loss-industry-grows-to-72-billion.

3. Grant M. Tinsley and Paul M. La Bounty, "Effects of intermittent fasting on body composition and clinical health markers in humans," *Nutrition Reviews* 73, no. 10 (October 2015): 661–674.

4. Moro et al., "Effects of eight weeks of time-restricted feeding (16/8) on basal metabolism, maximal strength, body composition, inflammation, and cardiovascular risk factors in resistance-trained males," 290.

5. Emily Gersema, "Scientifically designed fasting diet lowers risks for major diseases," USC News, February 16, 2017, https://news.usc.edu/116479/scientifically-designed-fasting-diet-lowers-risks-for-major-diseases/.

6. Satchin Panda, *The Circadian Code: Lose Weight, Supercharge Your Energy, and Transform Your Health from Morning to Midnight* (New York: Rodale Books, 2020).

7. Cribb, Julian, Surviving the 21st Century: *Humanity's Ten Great Challenges and How We Can Overcome Them* (Cham, Switzerland: Springer International Publishing, 2016).

8. Ameet Aggarwal, *Heal Your Body Cure Your Mind: Leaky Gut, Adrenal Fatigue, Liver Detox, Mental Health, Anxiety, Depression, Disease & Trauma, Mindfulness, Holistic Therapies, Diet, Nutrition & Food* (self-pub., CreateSpace, 2017).

9. Liaoliao Li, Zhi Wang, and Zhiyi Zuo, "Chronic Intermittent Fasting Improves Cognitive Functions and Brain Structures in Mice," *PloS One* 8, no. 6 (June 3, 2013): e66069.

10. Veerendra Kumar Madala Halagappa, Zhihong Guo, Michelle Pearson, Yasuji Matsuoka, Roy G. Cutler, Frank M. LaFerla, Mark P. Mattson, "Intermittent fasting and caloric restriction ameliorate age-related behavioral deficits in the triple-transgenic mouse model of Alzheimer's disease," Neurobiology of Disease, Volume 26, Issue 1, 2007, Pages 212-220, ISSN 0969-9961, https://doi.org/10.1016/j.nbd.2006.12.019.

11. Matthew Phillips, "Fasting as a Therapy in Neurological Disease," *Nutrients* 11, no. 10 (October 17, 2019): 2501, https://doi.org/10.3390/nu11102501.

12. Aliki I. Venetsanopoulou, Paraskevi V. Voulgari, and Alexandros A. Drosos, "Fasting mimicking diets: A literature review of their impact on inflammatory arthritis," *Mediterranean Journal of Rheumatology* 30, no. 4 (2019): 201–206.

13. Ali R Rahbar, Eisa Safavi, Maryam Rooholamini, Fateme Jaafari, Sadegh Darvishi, and Amin Rahbar, "Effects of Intermittent Fasting During Ramadan on Insulin-like Growth Factor-1, Interleukin 2, and Lipid Profile in Healthy Muslims," *International Journal of Preventive Medicine* 10, no. 7 (January 15, 2019); Rafael de Cabo and Mark P. Mattson, "Effects of Intermittent Fasting on Health, Aging, and Disease," *New England Journal of Medicine* 381, no. 26 (December 26, 2019): 2541–2551.

14. Martin P. Wegman, Michael H. Guo, Douglas M. Bennion, Meena N. Shankar, Stephen M. Chrzanowski, Leslie A. Goldberg, Jinze Xu et al., "Practicality of Intermittent Fasting in Humans and its Effect on Oxidative Stress and Genes Related to Aging and Metabolism," *Rejuvenation Research* 18, no. 2 (April 1, 2015): 162–172.

15. Mo'ez Al-Islam E. Faris, Safia Kacimi, Ref'at A. Al-Kurd, Mohammad A. Fararjeh, Yasser K. Bustanji, Mohammad K. Mohammad, and Mohammad L. Salem, "Intermittent Fasting During Ramadan Attenuates Proinflammatory Cytokines and Immune Cells in Healthy Subjects," *Nutrition Research* 32, no. 12 (December 2012): 947–955.

16. Catherine R. Marinac, Dorothy D. Sears, Loki Natarajan, Linda C. Gallo, Caitlin I. Breen, and Ruth E. Patterson, "Frequency and Circadian Timing of Eating May Influence Biomarkers of Inflammation and Insulin Resistance Associated with Breast Cancer Risk," *PloS One* 10, no. 8 (August 25, 2015): e0136240.

17. Wegman et al., "Practicality of Intermittent Fasting in Humans and its Effect on Oxidative Stress and Genes Related to Aging and Metabolism," 162–172.

18. Lee, C., Raffaghello, L., Brandhorst, S., Safdie, F. M., Bianchi, G., Martin-Montalvo, et al., "Fasting cycles retard growth of tumors and sensitize a range of cancer cell types to chemotherapy," *Science Translational Medicine* 4, no. 124 (March 27, 2012): 124ra27.

19. Faris et al., "Intermittent Fasting During Ramadan Attenuates Proinflammatory Cytokines and Immune Cells in Healthy Subjects," 947–955.

20. B. E. Engström, M. Öhrvall, M. Sundbom, L. Lind, and F. A. Karlsson, "Meal suppression of circulating ghrelin is normalized in obese individuals following gastric bypass surgery," *International Journal of Obesity* 31, no. 3 (August 22, 2006): 476–480.

21. Mohammed A. Alzoghaibi, Seithikurippu R. Pandi-Perumal, Munir M. Sharif, Ahmed S. BaHammam, "Diurnal Intermittent Fasting During Ramadan: The Effects on Leptin and Ghrelin Levels," *PloS One* 9, no.3 (March 17, 2014): e92214.

22. A. J. Carlson and F. Hoelzel, "Apparent Prolongation of the Life Span of Rats by Intermittent Fasting," *The Journal of Nutrition* 31 (March 1946): 363–375.

23. H. Sogawa and C. Kubo, "Influence of Short-Term Repeated Fasting on the Longevity of Female (NZB X NZW)F1 Mice," *Mechanisms of Ageing and Development* 115 no. 1–2 (May 18, 2000): 61–71.

24. Terra G. Arnason, Matthew W. Bowen, and Kerry D. Mansell, "Effects of Intermittent Fasting on Health Markers in Those with Type 2 Diabetes: A Pilot Study," *World Journal of Diabetes* 8, no. 4 (April 15, 2017): 154–164.

25. Adrienne R. Barnosky, Kristin K. Hoddy, Terry G. Unterman, and Krista A. Varady, "Intermittent Fasting vs Daily Calorie Restriction for Type 2 Diabetes Prevention: A Review of Human Findings," *Translational Research* 164 no. 4 (October 2014): 302–311.

26. Arnason et al., "Effects of Intermittent Fasting on Health Markers in Those With Type 2 Diabetes: A Pilot Study," 154–164.

27. Krista A. Varady, Surabhi Bhutani, Emily C. Church, and Monica C. Klempel, "Short-term Modified Alternate-Day Fasting: A Novel Dietary Strategy for Weight Loss and Cardioprotection in Obese Adults," *The American Journal of Clinical Nutrition* 90, no. 5 (November 2009): 1138–1143.

28. Abdullah Shehab, Abdishakur Abdulle, Awad El Issa, Jassim Al Suwaidi, and Nico Nagelkerke, "Favorable Changes in Lipid Profile: The Effects of Fasting After Ramadan," *PloS One* 7, no. 10 (2012): e47615.

29. Ruiqian Wan, Ismayil Ahmet, Martin Brown, Aiwu Cheng, Naomi Kamimura, Mark Talan, and Mark P. Mattson, "Cardioprotective Effect of Intermittent Fasting Is Associated with an Elevation of Adiponectin Levels in Rats," *The Journal of Nutritional Biochemistry* 21, no. 5 (May 2010): 413–417.

30. Rei Shibata, Noriyuki Ouchi, and Toyoaki Murohara, "Adiponectin and Cardiovascular Disease," *Circulation Journal* 73, no. 4 (2009), 608–614. https://doi.org/10.1253/circj.cj-09-0057

31. Edward Earle Purinton, *The Philosophy of Fasting* (Charleston, SC: BiblioLife, 2009).

32. Mark P. Mattson and Ruiqian Wan, "Beneficial Effects of Intermittent Fasting and Caloric Restriction on the Cardiovascular and Cerebrovascular Systems," *The Journal of Nutritional Biochemistry* 16, no. 3 (March 2005): 129–37; Nikos Kourtis and Nektarios Tavernarakis, "Cellular Stress Response Pathways and Ageing: Intricate Molecular Relationships," *The EMBO Journal* 30, no. 13 (May 17, 2011): 2520–2531.

33. Bob Rodgers, *101 Reasons to Fast* (Louisville, KY: Bob Rodgers Ministries, 1995), 52.

34. Louisa Lyon, "'All disease begins in the gut': was Hippocrates right?," *Brain* 141, no. 3 (March 2018): e20.

35. Mark Hyman, "How Good Gut Health Can Boost Your Immune System," EcoWatch, February 26, 2015, https://www.ecowatch .com/how-good-gut-health-can-boost-your-immune -system-1882013643.html.

36. Nair, P. M., & Khawale, P. G., "Role of therapeutic fasting in women's health: An overview," *Journal of Mid-Life Health*, 7(2), 61–64. https://doi.org/10.4103/0976-7800.185325.

37. John E. Morley, "Hormones and the Aging Process," *Journal of the American Geriatrics Society* 51, no. 7s (July 2003): S333–S337.

38. Ahmed, A., Saeed, F., Arshad, M. U., Afzaal, M., Imran, A., Ali, S. W., et al., "Impact of intermittent fasting on human health: an extended review of metabolic cascades," *International Journal of Food Properties* 21, no. 1 (January 6, 2019): 2700-2713.

39. Monica C. Klempel, Cynthia M. Kroeger, Surabhi Bhutani, John F. Trepanowski, and Krista A. Varady, "Intermittent Fasting Combined with Calorie Restriction Is Effective for Weight Loss and Cardio-Protection in Obese Women," *Nutrition Journal* 11, no. 98 (November 21, 2012).

40. Peter R. Kerndt, James L. Naughton, Charles E. Driscoll, and David A. Loxterkamp, "Fasting: The History, Pathophysiology and Complications," *The Western Journal of Medicine* 137, no. 5 (November 1982): 379–399.

41. Ho, K. Y., Veldhuis, J. D., Johnson, M. L., Furlanetto, R., Evans, W. S., Alberti, K. G., & Thorner, M. O. (1988), "Fasting enhances growth hormone secretion and amplifies the complex rhythms of growth hormone secretion in man," *The Journal of clinical investigation*, 81(4), 968-975.

PART 4: HOW AND WHEN TO FAST

1. Summar Habhab, Jane P. Sheldon, and Roger C. Loeb, "The Relationship Between Stress, Dietary Restraint, and Food Preferences in Women," *Appetite* 52, no. 2 (April 20089): 437–444.

2. David Perlmutter, *Brain Maker: The Power of Gut Microbes to Heal and Protect Your Brain—for Life* (New York: Little, Brown and Company, 2015).

3. Judith Matz and Ellen Frankel, *Beyond a Shadow of a Diet: The Comprehensive Guide to Treating Binge Eating Disorder, Compulsive Eating, and Emotional Overeating* (New York: Routledge, 2014).

4. Marcia Levin Pelchat, "Food Addiction in Humans," *The Journal of Nutrition* 139, no. 3 (March 2009): 620–622.

5. Susan M Himes and J. Kevin Thompson, "Fat Stigmatization in Television Shows and Movies: A Content Analysis," *Obesity*, 15, no. 3 (March 2007): 712–718.

6. Lexico, s.v. "drug," accessed June 9, 2020, https://www.lexico .com/en/definition/drug.

7. Ralph J. DiLeone, Jane R. Taylor, and Marina R. Picciotto, "The drive to eat: comparisons and distinctions between mechanisms of food reward and drug addiction," *Nature Neuroscience* 15, no. 10 (September 25, 2012): 1330.

8. Kent C Berridge, Chao-Yi Ho, Jocelyn M Richard, and Alexandra G DiFeliceantonio, "The Tempted Brain Eats: Pleasure and Desire Circuits in Obesity and Eating Disorders," *Brain Research* 1350 (September 2, 2010): 43–64.

9. Edward Leigh Gibson, "Emotional Influences on Food Choice: Sensory, Physiological and Psychological Pathways," *Physiology & Behavior* 89, no. 1 (August 30, 2006): 53–61.

10. Johannes Hebebrand, Özgür Albayrak, Roger Adan, Jochen Antel, Carlos Dieguez, Johannes de Jong, Gareth Leng et al., "'Eating Addiction,' Rather Than 'Food Addiction,' Better Captures Addictive-Like Eating Behavior," *Neuroscience & Biobehavioral Reviews* 47 (November 2014): 295–306.

11. Brian Wansink, *Mindless Eating: Why We Eat More Than We Think* (New York: Bantam Books, 2006).

12. Jennifer L. Placanica, Gavin J. Faunce, and Raymond Soames Job, "The effect of fasting on attentional biases for food and body shape/weight words in high and low eating disorder inventory scorers," *International Journal of Eating Disorders* 32, no. 1 (July 2002): 79–90.

13. John S. Allen, *The Omnivorous Mind: Our Evolving Relationship with Food* (Cambridge, MA: Harvard University Press, 2012).

14. "About EWG's Shopper's Guide to Pesticides in Produce," Environmental Working Group, accessed June 9, 2020, https://www.ewg.org/foodnews/about.php.

15. "Clean Fifteen," Environmental Working Group, accessed June 9, 2020, https://www.ewg.org/foodnews/clean-fifteen.php; "Dirty Dozen," Environmental Working Group, accessed June 9, 2020, https://www.ewg.org/foodnews/dirty-dozen.php.

16. *Merriam-Webster*, s.v. "satiety," accessed June 9, 2020, https://www.merriam-webster.com/dictionary/satiety.

17. Hendrik Jan Smit, E. Katherine Kemsley, Henri S. Tapp, and C. Jeya K. Henry, "Does Prolonged Chewing Reduce Food Intake? Fletcherism Revisited," *Appetite* 57 no. 1 (August 2011): 295–298.

18. John A. Bargh, Annette Lee-Chai, Kimberly Barndollar, Peter M. Gollwitzer, and Roman Trötschel, "The Automated Will: Nonconscious Activation and Pursuit of Behavioral Goals," *Journal of Personality and Social Psychology* 81, no. 6 (December 2001): 1014–1027.

19. Edwin A. Locke, "Motivation through conscious goal setting," *Applied & Preventive Psychology* 5, no. 2 (1996): 117–124.

20. Christie L. K. Kawada, Gabriele Oettingen, Peter M. Gollwitzer, and John A. Bargh, "The Projection of Implicit and Explicit Goals," *Journal of Personality and Social Psychology* 86, no. 4 (April 2004): 545–559.

21. David Zinczenko, *The 8-Hour Diet: Watch the Pounds Disappear Without Watching What You Eat!* (New York, Rodale, 2013), xi.

Part 5: FASTING FAQS

1. Janet Polivy, "Psychological Consequences of Food Restriction," *Journal of the American Dietetic Association* 96, no. 6 (June 1996): 589–592; Janet Polivy, "The effects of behavioral inhibition: Integrating internal cues, cognition, behavior, and affect," *Psychological Inquiry* 9, no. 3 (1998): 181–204; A. V. Kurpad, S. Muthayya, and M. Vaz, "Consequences of Inadequate Food Energy and Negative Energy Balance in Humans," *Public Health Nutrition*, 8, no. 7A (October 2005): 1053–1076.

2. Sushil Kumar and Gurcharan Kaur, "Intermittent Fasting Dietary Restriction Regimen Negatively Influences Reproduction in Young Rats: A Study of Hypothalamo-Hypophysial-Gonadal Axis," *PloS One* 8, no. 1 (2013): e52416.

3. Kumar et al., "Intermittent Fasting Dietary Restriction Regimen Negatively Influences Reproduction in Young Rats."

4. Amy Shah, "The Secret to Intermittent Fasting for Women," Dr. Axe, May 22, 2016, https://draxe.com/nutrition/intermittent-fasting-women/.

5. "Type 2 diabetes reversed by losing fat from pancreas," *ScienceDaily*, September 13, 2017, https://www.sciencedaily.com/releases/2017/09/170913084432.htm.

6. B. Claustrat and J. Leston, "Melatonin: Physiological effects in humans," *Neurosurgery* 6, no. 2–3 (April – June 2015), 77–84.

7. Koenraad Philippaert, Andy Pironet, Margot Mesuere, William Sones, Laura Vermeiren, Sara Kerselaers et al., "Steviol glycosides enhance pancreatic beta-cell function and taste sensation by potentiation of TRPM5 channel activity," *Nature Communications* 8, no. 1 (March 31, 2017): 1–16.

PART 6: SMART FASTING TOOLS

1. Mahmoud M. Suhail, Weijuan Wu, Amy Cao, Fadee G. Mondalek, Kar-Ming Fung, Pin-Tsen Shih, Yu-Ting Fang et al., "Boswellia Sacra Essential Oil Induces Tumor Cell-Specific Apoptosis and Suppresses Tumor Aggressiveness in Cultured Human Breast Cancer Cells," *BMC Complementary and Alternative Medicine* 11 (December 15, 2011): 129.

2. Rashmi Choudhary, K. P. Mishra, and C. Subramanyam, "Prevention of isoproterenol-induced cardiac hypertrophy by eugenol, an antioxidant," *Indian Journal of Clinical Biochemistry* 21, no. 2 (September 2006): 107–113.

3. S. Katsuyama, H. Mizoguchi, H. Kuwahata, T. Komatsu, K. Nagaoka, H. Nakamura, G. Bagetta et al., "Involvement of Peripheral Cannabinoid and Opioid Receptors in β-Caryophyllene-Induced Antinociception," *European Journal of Pain* 17, no. 5 (May 2013): 664–675; Adriano Guimarães-Santos, Diego Siqueira Santos, Ijair Rogério Santos, Rafael Rodrigues Lima, Antonio Pereira, Lucinewton Silva de Moura, Raul Nunes Carvalho Jr. et al., "Copaiba Oil-Resin Treatment Is Neuroprotective and Reduces Neutrophil Recruitment and Microglia Activation after Motor Cortex Excitotoxic Injury," *Evidence-Based Complementary and Alternative Medicine* (2012); Amine Bahi, Shamma Al Mansouri, Elyazia Al Memari, Mouza Al Ameri, Syed M Nurulain, and Shreesh Ojha, "β-Caryophyllene, a CB2 Receptor Agonist Produces Multiple Behavioral Changes Relevant to Anxiety and Depression in Mice," *Physiology & Behavior* 135 (August 2014): 119–124; Shamma Al Mansouri, Shreesh Ojha, Elyazia Al Maamari, Mouza Al Ameri, Syed M Nurulain, and Amine Bahi, "The Cannabinoid Receptor 2 Agonist, β-Caryophyllene, Reduced

8. Gregory Traversy and Jean-Philippe Chaput, "Alcohol Consumption and Obesity: An Update," *Current Obesity Reports* 4, no. 1 (March 2015): 122–130.

9. de Cabo et al., "Effects of Intermittent Fasting on Health, Aging, and Disease," 2541–2551.

10. Fernando M. Safdie, Tanya Dorff, David Quinn, Luigi Fontana, Min Wei, Changhan Lee, Pinchas Cohen, and Valter D. Longo, "Fasting and cancer treatment in humans: A case series report," *Aging* 1, no. 12 (December 31, 2009): 988.

11. R. Sichieri, J. E. Everhart, and H. Roth, "A prospective study of hospitalization with gallstone disease among women: role of dietary factors, fasting period, and dieting," *American Journal of Public Health* 81, no. 7 (July 1991): 880–884.

12. Rima Solianik, Laura Žlibinaitė, Margarita Drozdova-Statkevičienė, and Artūras Sujeta, "Forty-eight-hour fasting declines mental flexibility but improves balance in overweight and obese older women," *Physiology & Behavior* 223 (September 1, 2020): 112995.

13. Anita Boelen, Wilmar Maarten Wiersinga, and Eric Fliers, "Fasting-induced Changes in the Hypothalamus-Pituitary-Thyroid Axis," *Thyroid: Official Journal of the American Thyroid Association* 18 no. 2 (February 2008): 123–129.

14. Fontana, L., Klein, S., Holloszy, J. O., & Premachandra, B. N. (2006). Effect of long-term calorie restriction with adequate protein and micronutrients on thyroid hormones. *The Journal of clinical endocrinology and metabolism*, 91(8), 3232–3235. https://doi.org/10.1210/jc.2006-0328

Voluntary Alcohol Intake and Attenuated Ethanol-Induced Place Preference and Sensitivity in Mice," *Pharmacology, Biochemistry, and Behavior* 124 (September 2014): 260–268.

4. P. Agrawal, V. Rai, and R. B. Singh, "Randomized Placebo-Controlled, Single Blind Trial of Holy Basil Leaves in Patients with Noninsulin-Dependent Diabetes Mellitus," *Journal of Clinical Pharmacology and Therapeutics* 34, no. 9 (September 1996): 406–409.

5. A. T. Peana, P. S. D'Aquila, F. Panin, G. Serra, P. Pippia, and M. D. L. Moretti, "Anti-inflammatory Activity of Linalool and Linalyl Acetate Constituents of Essential Oils," *Phytomedicine* 9, no. 8 (December 2002): 721–726; "Linalyl acetate," National Library of Medicine, accessed June 9, 2020, https://pubchem.ncbi.nlm.nih.gov/compound/Linalyl-acetate.

6. Hichem Sebai, Slimen Selmi, Kais Rtibi, Abdelaziz Souli, Najoua Gharbi, and Mohsen Sakly, "Lavender (Lavandula Stoechas L.) Essential Oils Attenuate Hyperglycemia and Protect Against Oxidative Stress in Alloxan-Induced Diabetic Rats," *Lipids in Health and Disease* 12 (December 28, 2013): 189.

7. Kei Sato, Sabine Krist, and Gerhard Buchbauer, "Antimicrobial effect of vapours of geraniol, (R)-(-)-linalool, terpineol, gamma-terpinene and 1,8-cineole on airborne microbes using an airwasher," *Flavour and Fragrance Journal* 22, no. 5 (September/October 2007): 435–43; F. A. Santos, V. S. Rao," Antiinflammatory and Antinociceptive Effects of 1,8-cineole a Terpenoid Oxide Present in Many Plant Essential Oils." *Phytotherapy Research* 14, no. 4 (June 2000): 240–244.

8. Mark Moss and Lorraine Oliver, "Plasma 1,8-cineole correlates with cognitive performance following exposure to rosemary essential oil aroma," *Therapeutic Advances in Psychopharmacology* 2, no. 3 (June 2012): 103–113.

9. Joerg Hucklenbroich, Rebecca Klein, Bernd Neumaier, Rudolf Graf, Gereon Rudolf Fink, Michael Schroeter, and Maria Adele Rueger, "Aromatic-turmerone Induces Neural Stem Cell Proliferation in Vitro and in Vivo," *Stem Cell Research & Therapy* 5, no. 4 (September 26, 2014): 100; Marie-Hélène Teiten, Serge Eifes, Mario Dicato, and Marc Diederich, "Curcumin-the Paradigm of a Multi-Target Natural Compound With Applications in Cancer Prevention and Treatment," *Toxins* 2, no. 1 (January 2010): 128–162; Sun Young Park, Mei Ling Jin, Young Hun Kim, Young Hee Kim, and Sang Joon Lee, "Anti-inflammatory Effects of Aromatic-Turmerone Through Blocking of NF-κB, JNK, and p38 MAPK Signaling Pathways in Amyloid β-Stimulated Microglia," *International Immunopharmacology* 14, no. 1 (September 2012): 13–20.

10. Pete J. Cox and Kieran Clarke, "Acute nutritional ketosis: implications for exercise performance and metabolism," *Extreme Physiology and Medicine* 3 (2014): 17.

11. Ai-Ling Lin, Wei Zhang, Xiaoli Gao, and Lora Watts, "Caloric Restriction Increases Ketone Bodies Metabolism and Preserves Blood Flow in Aging Brain," *Neurobiology of Aging* 36, no. 7 (July 2015): 2296–2303.

12. Philippe J. M. Pinckaers, Tyler A. Churchward-Venne, David Bailey, and Luc J. C. van Loon, "Ketone Bodies and Exercise Performance: The Next Magic Bullet or Merely Hype?" *Sports Medicine* (Auckland, N.Z.) 47, no. 3 (March 2017), 383–391.

13. Andrew J. Murray, Nicholas S. Knight, Mark A. Cole, Lowri E. Cochlin, Emma Carter, Kirill Tchabanenko, Tica Pichulik et al., "Novel Ketone Diet Enhances Physical and Cognitive Performance," *FASEB Journal: Official Publication of the Federation of American Societies for Experimental Biology* 30, no. 12 (2016): 4021–4032.

14. Mark Evans, Karl E. Cogan, and Brendan Egan, "Metabolism of Ketone Bodies During Exercise and Training: Physiological Basis for Exogenous Supplementation," *The Journal of Physiology* 595, no. 9 (May 1, 2017): 2857–2871.

15. Darren E. R. Warburton, Crystal Whitney Nicol, and Shannon S. D. Bredin, "Health benefits of physical activity: the evidence," *CMAJ: Canadian Medical Association Journal* 174, no. 6 (March 14, 2006): 801–809.

16. Ahimsa Porter Sumchai, "The Exercise Prescription Therapeutic Applications of Exercise and Physical Activity," *Journal of Novel Physiotherapies* 3 (June 10, 2013): 148–153.

17. "Meditation in Depth," National Center for Complementary and Integrative Health, updated June 9, 2020, https://www .nccih.nih.gov/health/meditation-in-depth.

18. Susan L. Smalley and Diana Winston, *Fully Present: The Science, Art, and Practice of Mindfulness* (Philadelphia, PA: Da Capo Press, 2010).

19. D. P. Wirth, "The Significance of Belief and Expectancy Within the Spiritual Healing Encounter," *Social Science & Medicine* 41, no. 2 (July 1995): 249–260.

20. David S. Weigle, Patricia A. Breen, Colleen C. Matthys, Holly S. Callahan, Kaatje E. Meeuws, Verna R. Burden, and Jonathan Q. Purnell, "A High-Protein Diet Induces Sustained Reductions in Appetite, Ad Libitum Caloric Intake, and Body Weight Despite Compensatory Changes in Diurnal Plasma Leptin and Ghrelin Concentrations," *The American Journal of Clinical Nutrition* 82, no. 1 (July 2005): 41–48.

21. Jordan L. Hawkins and Paul L. Durham, "Enriched Chicken Bone Broth as a Dietary Supplement Reduces Nociception and Sensitization Associated with Prolonged Jaw Opening," *Journal of Oral & Facial Pain and Headache* 32, no. 2 (March

6, 2018): 208–215; Faris et al., "Intermittent Fasting During Ramadan Attenuates Proinflammatory Cytokines and Immune Cells in Healthy Subjects," 947–955.

22. E. Proksch, D. Segger, J. Degwert, M. Schunck, V. Zague, and S. Oesser, "Oral Supplementation of Specific Collagen Peptides Has Beneficial Effects on Human Skin Physiology: A Double-Blind, Placebo-Controlled Study," *Skin Pharmacology and Physiology* 27, no. 1 (2014): 47–55.

About the Authors

JORDAN RUBIN

New York Times best-selling author

Cofounder, Ancient Nutrition

Jordan Rubin is one of America's most recognized and respected natural health experts and is the *New York Times* best-selling author of *The Maker's Diet*, as well as twenty-five additional titles, including *Essential Oils: Ancient Medicine*.

An eco-entrepreneur, author, and lecturer on health and nutrition, Jordan has shared a message of health and hope on five continents and in forty-six states in the United States.

Jordan is the founder of Garden of Life, the leading whole-food nutritional supplement company, and Beyond Organic, a vertically integrated organic food, beverage, and dietary supplement manufacturer. Jordan has formulated hundreds of dietary supplements, functional foods, and beverages, including many number-one top sellers in the Healthy Foods channel.

In 2016, along with cofounder Dr. Josh Axe, Jordan launched Ancient Nutrition, a company that brings the principles of ancient nutrition to the modern world.

Jordan is the founder of Heal the Planet Farm, a regenerative permaculture retreat located in Missouri's Ozark mountains within the four thousand–acre Beyond Organic Ranch.

Jordan and his beautiful wife, Nicki, are the parents of six wonderful children.

DR. JOSH AXE, DNM, DC, CNS

Cofounder, Ancient Nutrition

Dr. Josh Axe is a doctor of natural medicine, doctor of chiropractic, clinical nutritionist, and creator of DrAxe.com, one of the world's largest natural health websites.

Dr. Axe is a best-selling author of the ground-breaking health books *Eat Dirt*, *Keto Diet*, and *The Collagen Diet*.

A physician for many professional athletes, Dr. Axe began working with the Wellness Advisory Council in 2009 and traveled to the 2012 Games in London to work with Team USA athletes. Dr. Axe is an expert in digestive health, functional medicine, natural remedies, and dietary strategies for healing. He has been featured on leading television networks and programs including *The Dr. Oz Show*, CBS, and NBC and is the host of three PBS specials.

Dr Josh Axe resides in Nashville, Tennessee, with his wife, Dr. Chelsea Axe, and their daughter.

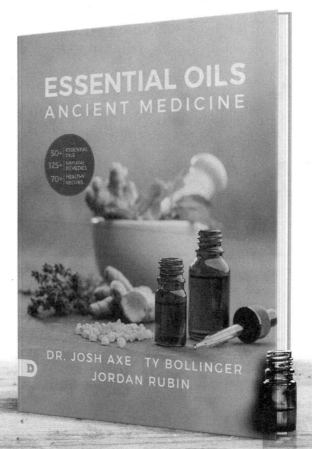

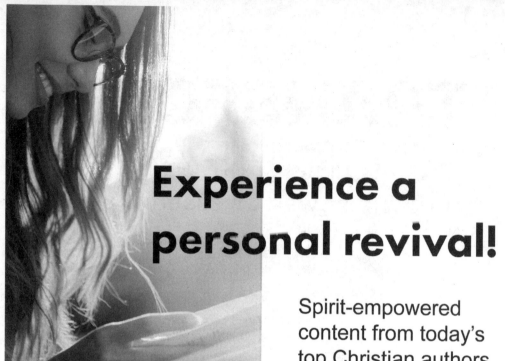
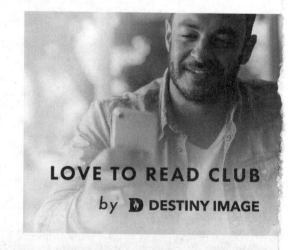

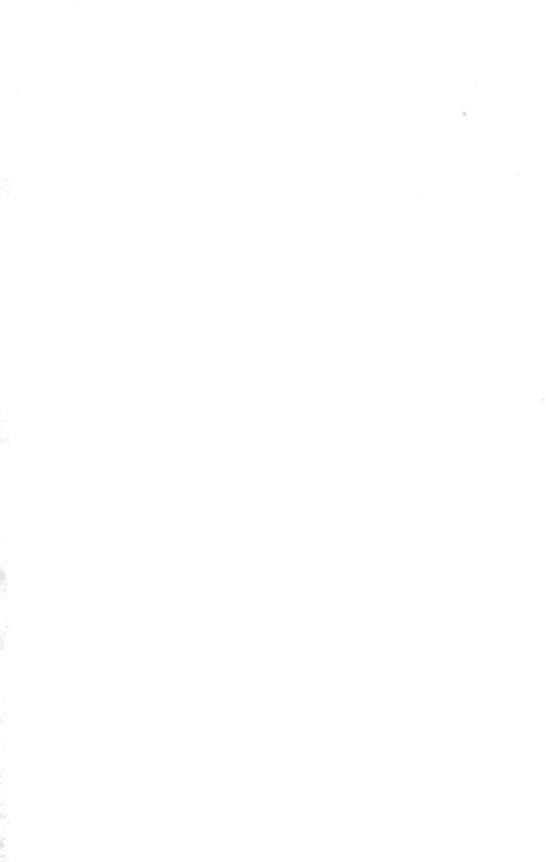